Sue Corbett

INTRODUCTION TO SPINE SURGERY

ESSENTIALS FOR ORP, FELLOWS, AND RESIDENTS

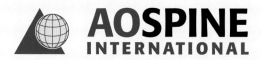

Sue Corbett

INTRODUCTION TO SPINE SURGERY

ESSENTIALS FOR ORP, FELLOWS, AND RESIDENTS

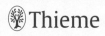

Foreword by John K Webb

Design and layout: Sandro Isler, nougat GmbH, CH-4056 Basel
Illustrations: nougat GmbH, CH-4056 Basel
Production: AO Publishing, CH-8600 Dübendorf

Library of Congress Cataloging-in-Publication Data is available from the publisher.

Printed in Switzerland

ISBN 3-13-143351-5
ISBN 1-58890-469-5

CONTRIBUTORS

EDITOR

Sue Corbett, RN
Spinal Theatre Sister
The Center for Spinal Surgery
University Hospital
Queens Medical Centre
Nottingham, UK

AUTHORS

John R Andrews, MB, BCh, FRCS
(Trauma & Orthopedics)
Consultant Spinal Surgeon
The Royal Orthopedic Hospital
Birmingham, UK

Debra Beer
Senior Clinical Physiologist
(Neurophysiology)
University Hospital
Queens Medical Centre
Nottingham, UK

Andrew Clarke, BSc (Hons), MBBS, MRCS
Specialist Registrar (Trauma & Orthopedics)
Royal Cornwall Hospital
Truro
Cornwall, UK

Brian JC Freeman, MB, BCh, BAO, FRCS
(Trauma & Orthopedics)
Consultant Spinal Surgeon
The Centre for Spinal Surgery
University Hospital
Queens Medical Centre
Nottingham, UK

Michele Goodwin, RN
Main Theatres, Recovery Team
University Hospital
Queens Medical Centre
Nottingham, UK

Angela Hallworth, RN
Main Theatres, Recovery Team
University Hospital
Queens Medical Centre
Nottingham, UK

Hayley Johnson, RN
Main Theatres, Recovery Team
University Hospital
Queens Medical Centre
Nottingham, UK

Alwyn Jones, MB, BCh, BSc, (Hons), MSc,
FRCS (Trauma & Orthopedics)
Consultant Spinal Surgeon
University Hospital of Wales
Heath Park
Cardiff, UK

Ruth Knight, RN
Main Theatres, Recovery Team
University Hospital
Queens Medical Centre
Nottingham, UK

Michael JH McCarthy, BMedSci, BMBS
(Hons), MRCS (Eng)
Spinal Research Fellow
The Centre for Spinal Surgery
University Hospital
Queens Medical Centre
Nottingham, UK

Patrick J McKenna MB, BS, FRCS
(Trauma & Orthopedics)
Consultant Spinal Surgeon
Royal Berkshire Hospital
Reading, UK

Clare VJ Morgan-Hough, MB, BS,
BSc (Hons), FRACS
(Trauma & Orthopedics)
Consultant Spinal Surgeon
Robert Jones and Agnes Hunt
District Hospital
Oswestry, UK

Robert C Mulholland, Professor,
MB, BS, D Obst, RCOG, FRCS
Consultant Spinal Surgon
Emeritus Nottingham University Hospital
Special Professor in Trauma
and Orthopedics
The Centre for Spinal Surgery
University Hospital
Queens Medical Centre
Nottingham, UK

Jabir Nagaria, MMBS, FRCS (Neurosurgery)
Locum Consultant Spinal Surgeon
The Centre for Spinal Surgery
University Hospital
Queens Medical Centre
Nottingham, UK

Helen Nelson, RN
Main Theatres, Recovery Team
University Hospital
Queens Medical Centre
Nottingham, UK

Carmel Nosworthy, RN
Main Theatres, Recovery Team
University Hospital
Queens Medical Centre
Nottingham, UK

Robert W Nowicki, MB, BS, FRCA
Consultant Anesthetist
Anesthetic Department
University Hospital
Queens Medical Centre
Nottingham, UK

Mike O'Malley, BSc (Hons), MB, BCh, MSc,
FRCS (Trauma & Orthopedics)
Consultant Trauma & Orthopedic Surgeon
North Cheshire Hospitals NHS Trust
Warrington
Cheshire, UK,

Janine Roulston, RN
Main Theatres, Recovery Team
University Hospital
Queens Medical Centre
Nottingham, UK

Toni Swaby, EN, RN
Main Theatres, Recovery Team
University Hospital
Queens Medical Centre
Nottingham, UK

Sue Ward, SEN
Main Theatres, Recovery Team
University Hospital
Queens Medical Centre
Nottingham, UK

REVIEWERS

Robert C Watkins, IV, MD
Spinal Surgeon
Los Angeles Spinal Surgery Center
Los Angeles, CA, USA

Christina Zarifova, RN
Main Theatres, Recovery Team
University Hospital
Queens Medical Centre
Nottingham, UK

Paul M Arnold, MD, FACS
Professor of Neurosurgery
Director Spinal Cord Injury Center
University of Kansas Medical Center
Kansas City, MO, US

Helton Defino, MD
Hospital das Clinicas da Faculdade de
Medicina de Ribeirao Preto USP
Campus Universitário
J Canadá – Ribeirão Preto
São Paulo, BR

Claudio Lamartina, MD, Professor
Chief of Spine Surgery Departement
Istituto Ortopedico Galeazzi
Milano, IT

Richard Williams, FRACS, MBBS
Reference Centre Director
Princess Alexandra Hospital
Brisbane, QLD, AU

OTHER CONTRIBUTORS

Michael E Janssen, DO
Chairman of Board
Spine Education & Research Institute
University of Colorado
Center for Spinal Disorders
Denver, CO, US

John K O'Dowd, MD, FRCS, MBBS
Director of Spine Surgery
Guy's and St Thomas Hospitals
London, UK

John Pinsent
1 Arlington House
The Park
Nottingham, UK

John K Webb, MD, FRCS
Consultant Spinal Surgeon
Chief of Spine Unit
University Hospital
Queens Medical Centre
Nottingham, UK

FOREWORD

It is a double pleasure for me to write the foreword to this book.

First, I have known Sue Corbett, the book's Editor-in-Chief since the opening of our Spinal Unit at the Queens Medical Centre, Nottingham, in October 1993. Sue, as a member of our operating room personnel (ORP) is truly a rare breed in that she has chosen to specialize in spine management.

In fact, Sue has been instrumental in developing the quality of the spinal operating rooms as well as many of our spine protocols. There is little doubt that much of the expertise and knowledge of our ORP is largely due to the enthusiasm and quality of our senior staff and in particular Sue.

On a wider note, the book also marks a first for AOSpine, the spine organization within the AO Foundation. I am proud to say that I was directly involved in the creation of AOSpine, and it was always my personal vision for our "spine" community to grow beyond the founding surgeons, and to embrace all key members of the spine care team.

Sue can take pride that this AOSpine's first true venture into providing direct support for ORP. I am confident that this book will be of great value to ORP and will be a good foundation to new services from AOSpine directed to this vital group.

Actually, I am doing a disservice to the book; although it began as an introduction of spine surgery for ORP, it has developed beyond its original scope. I can therefore also strongly recommend it for fellows and residents considering entering the field of spine surgery.

My last words are simple, enjoy this book, and enjoy spine!

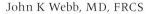

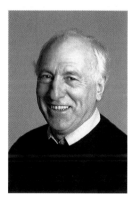

John K Webb, MD, FRCS

PREFACE

I have been a member of the operating room personnel (ORP) team at the Centre for Spinal Surgery, University Hospital, Queens Medical Centre, Nottingham, UK, since it opened its doors in October 1993, integrating the orthopedic spine services to one site, under the direction of Mr John K Webb and his colleagues Prof Robert C Mulholland and Miss Heather G Prince.

This book has developed from an idea I had while developing my skills in the spinal ORs during the past twelve years. When I entered this specialty I had limited knowledge on the subject, so it was an entirely new learning environment for me. Although there were many textbooks for ORP, none related specifically to orthopedic spine surgery, and I always felt that a straightforward reference book for operating room staff would be invaluable, hence my attempt to gather together the knowledge and skills presently available in this area in one setting.

The aim of this book is to offer guidance and foster a wider knowledge and understanding of the subject, thus enabling the multidisciplinary surgical team to enhance their skills and address the many challenges unique to each patient during their preoperative care. I hope this book will help other teams in the future, as the information it contains has never before been compiled in this manner. It is intended to provide an

outline of spine surgery for the multidisciplinary team, with particular emphasis for the ORP and spine surgery residents that are primarily concerned with providing care for these patients. Time to learn about individual specialties is always in short supply for any team member in today's OR setting. With this in mind, I have tried to keep the style of the book clear and concise, while still retaining the key information required for addressing the needs of spinal patients throughout their preoperative, intraoperative, and postoperative caring pathways.

Spine surgery has advanced dramatically over the past twelve years. Implants are being constantly biomechanically improved to meet the needs of surgical management, meaning that surgical treatment of the injured, painful, and deformed spine may be addressed promptly and effectively to allow early mobilization of the patient.

All patients have certain common care needs; however, the detailed attention to these needs can vary not just from country to country but from hospital to hospital. Because of this variation this book can only aim to outline the general principles, equipment, and surgical options used to treat the patient in this complex matrix of care.

While this book addresses the patient's journey through the OR, it does not discuss specific implant systems. Implants do have a very important role to play, and there is a wide variety available on the market, but the selection of implants is a matter of surgical preference and thus outside the scope of this book.

I wish to express my sincere thanks to all who have advised and supported me in reaching the goal of bringing this book together over the past twelve months. Very special thanks must go to the contributors, who have found time in their very busy schedules to complete their excellent chapters.

Over the last twelve years I have worked with many people within the spinal family; consultant spine surgeons both past and present, spine fellows both from the UK and from overseas, who have successfully completed fellowships at Nottingham, a dedicated OR spinal team, and Jim Hegarty and Ruth Friesem who supported me in the early years. I would therefore like to dedicate this book to all the team members who have helped me gain the knowledge and expertise I hold today. Without their encouragement and support this book would never have been written.

I am indebted to AO Publishing and AOSpine International who believed in what I wanted to produce. Finally, a very special thank you must go to Cristina Lusti at AO Publishing for all her help and support as my book coordinator.

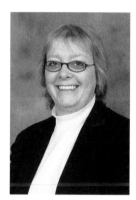

S. Corbett

Sue Corbett, RN

ACKNOWLEDGMENTS

I would like to acknowledge my thanks to the following people, who contributed towards this book.

Special thanks and support to the reviewers who during their own busy schedule found time to review this book and to feedback very wise and expert advice to me. All their input was taken into account and changes made on their recommendations. Thanks to: Paul M Arnold and his team (Andrew Engelhardt, Lisa Lampe, Lisa Reiman, Kristin Deere), Helton Defino, Claudio Lamartina, Richard Williams, John Pinsent, and Mike Janssen.

I am also grateful to the following people, whose expert knowledge within their field also played a part in helping contributors in their chapters: John O'Dowd, John Webb, Heather Prince, YH Yau, Lee Breakwell, James F Hegarty, Angela McDonnel, David Pinnock, Margaret Stone, Kate Britton, Dawn Hyde, and Karen Thornley.

Sue Corbett

TABLE OF CONTENTS

GENERAL KNOWLEDGE
FOR SPINE SURGERY

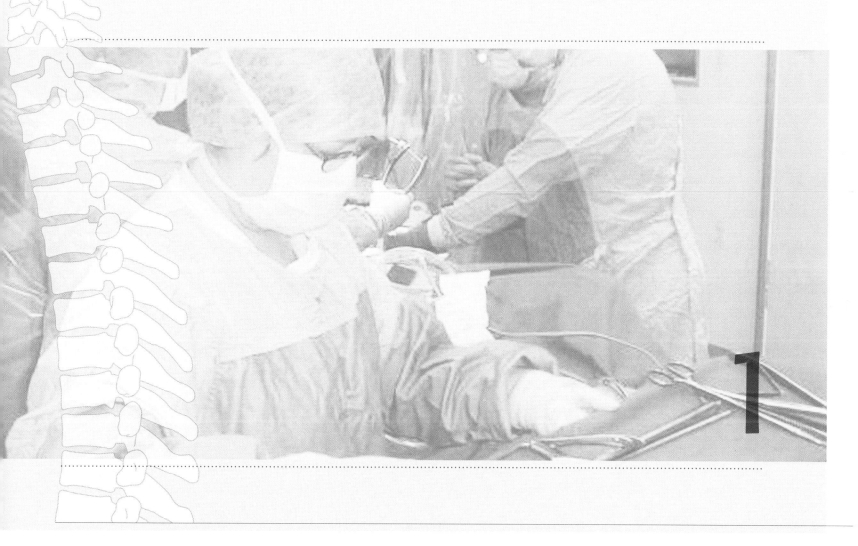

1

1   GENERAL KNOWLEDGE FOR SPINE SURGERY

1.1   ANATOMY OF THE SPINE

1   PLANES AND DIRECTIONS

An operating room team must be able to understand the terminology used by the medical team during surgery in relation to the human anatomy. Knowledge of planes and directions is an essential element required by all team members in order to speak a common language (**Fig 1.1-1**).

- Anterior
  Situated towards the front of the patient. This indicates that the incision will be via the throat, chest, or abdomen.
- Posterior
  Situated towards the back of the patient. This indicates that the incision will be down the back of the spine and the surgeon should indicate at which level.
- Cranial
  Situated towards the head of the patient.
  This indicates the surgeon is referring to the level above or another segment above.

- Caudal
  Situated towards the feet of the patient. This indicates the surgeon is referring to the lower levels or segments.
- Medial
  Refers to the midline.
- Lateral
  Refers to the side away from the midline.
- Coronal plane
  Divides the body into the anterior and posterior.
- Sagittal plane
  Divides the body into right and left sides.
- Axial plane
  Divides the body into top and bottom. This is a view from above or parallel to the main axis and lies at 90° to each of the other planes.

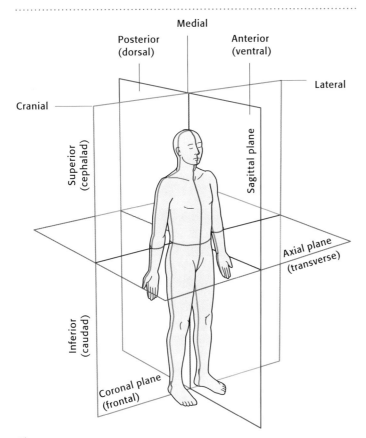

Medial

Posterior
(dorsal)

Anterior
(ventral)

Lateral

Cranial

Superior
(cephalad)

Sagittal plane

Axial plane
(transverse)

Inferior
(caudad)

Coronal plane
(frontal)

Fig 1.1-1
Planes and directions.

2   FUNCTION OF THE SPINE

The vertebral column construction consists of vertebrae, discs, ligaments, and muscles. All have a part to play in providing us with some stability plus mobility, and letting us function in the upright position, thus allowing various activities. The vertebrae are ring-like structures that provide bony protection to the spinal cord, meninges, and associated vessels. Their segmental nature allows flexibility. As a column, the spine provides support to the torso at the thoracic levels, and together with the ribs prevents compression to the heart, lungs, and major vessels. The load-bearing ability at this level is increased threefold. The discs are fibrocartilagenous and act as a shock absorber against axial load, allowing weight distribution. The ligamentous and muscular structures help maintain stability of the spine like the guy rope of a tent.

3   CURVES OF THE SPINE

The two most important profiles of the spine are the sagittal plus the coronal planes.

The spine is viewed in two ways: the lateral and posterior aspect. This terminology is heard constantly during spine surgery. A requirement in all spinal procedures is a plain anterior and posterior x-ray; however, magnetic resonance imaging (MRI) and computed tomography (CT) are used to give a more detailed view of bone and tissues (see chapter 1.2 Imaging of the spine).

In the posterior view (coronal profile), the spine appears symmetrical and straight (**Fig 1.1-2**). In the lateral view (sagittal profile), it consists of four natural curves (**Fig 1.1-3**), two lordosis and two kyphosis (**Fig 1.1-4**). These curves are not present at birth, but evolve as the infant develops. The cervical and lumbar spine curves are referred to as a lordosis or a lordotic curve; the convexity of the curve is positioned anteriorly. The thoracic and sacral spine curves are referred to as a kyphosis or a kyphotic curve; the concavity of the curve is positioned anteriorly.

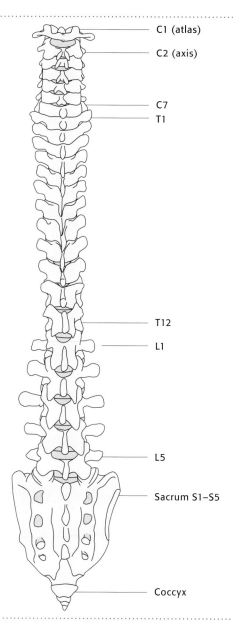

C1 (atlas)
C2 (axis)
C7
T1
T12
L1
L5
Sacrum S1–S5
Coccyx

Fig 1.1-2
Posterior view of the spinal column.

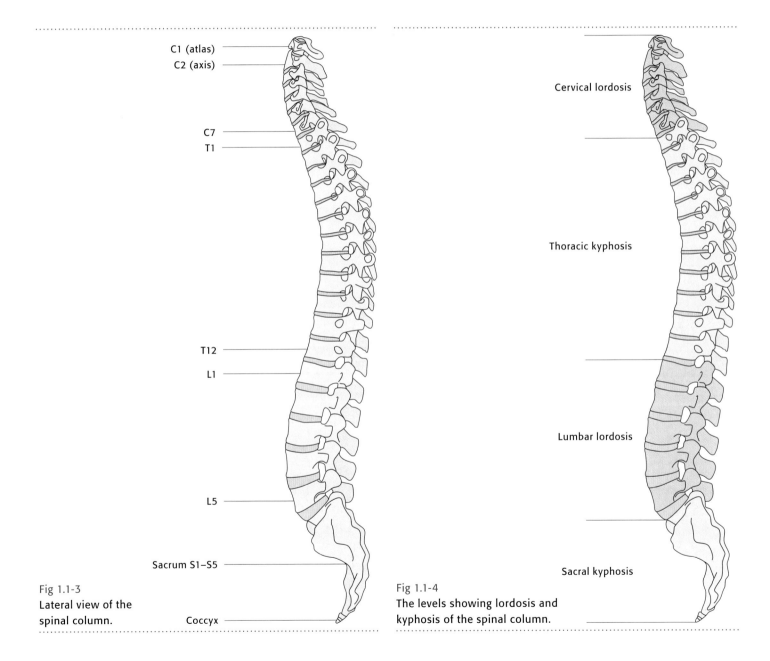

C1 (atlas)
C2 (axis)

C7
T1

T12

L1

L5

Sacrum S1–S5

Coccyx

Fig 1.1-3
Lateral view of the
spinal column.

Cervical lordosis

Thoracic kyphosis

Lumbar lordosis

Sacral kyphosis

Fig 1.1-4
The levels showing lordosis and
kyphosis of the spinal column.

4   LEVELS OF THE SPINE

Defining levels before and during surgery is paramount to the success of the procedure. The adult spine is on average 70 cm long, with the bony column divided into five main regions: cervical, thoracic, lumbar, sacrum, and coccyx.

Although there is similarity between each of the five regions there are distinctive features that differentiate one region from another. The column is made up of 33 different vertebrae and denoted as:

- Cervical: C1–C7
- Thoracic: T1–T12
- Lumbar: L1–L5
- Sacrum: S1–S5
- Coccyx: C1–C4

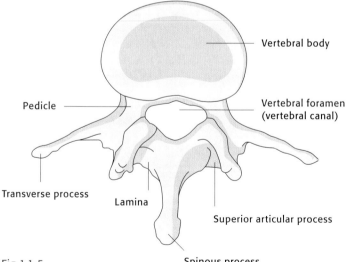

Pedicle

Vertebral body

Vertebral foramen (vertebral canal)

Transverse process

Lamina

Superior articular process

Spinous process

Fig 1.1-5
The seven sections of a typical vertebra.

5   VERTEBRAL ANATOMY

Shared features can be found in the vertebrae, vertebral body, and the posterior arch. Between the body and the arch is the vertebral foramen, which houses the spinal cord. The seven sections of a typical vertebra can be seen in **Fig 1.1-5**.

The body is the largest section, which bears 80% of the loads applied to the spine; on both the superior and inferior surfaces it is flat where the disc is situated and is composed of cancellous bone with a dense surrounding of cortical bone. The spongy cancellous section is highly vascular, and is a storage space for nutrients and blood cells; the cortical section is a structural support for the main body.

The posterior arch takes on a different form, which is made up of five sections:

- Pedicle
  There are two, one at each side of the body. They are short, thick cylinders of bone that project posteriorly. The function of these structures is to form a bridge between the body and the posterior arch.

- Lamina
  The left and right laminae consist of a broad shield of cortical bone that extends from the pedicles and completes the arch; the function is to shelter the cord.

- Spinous process
  Projects posteriorly, situated between the laminae, at the point of which they fuse. It is the most superficial segment of the spine when viewed from behind.

- Transverse processes
  The left and right ones extend laterally from the junction

of the lamina and pedicle. Both these processes are the attachment points for muscles, which allow movement of the spine, and ligaments, which stabilize the spine.

- Articular processes
  There are four processes, two superior and two transverse. Two project superiorly and two project inferiorly from the junction between the pedicle and lamina. The articulating surfaces of these processes are called facets and are covered with hyaline cartilage.

The vertebrae are stacked on top of one another, allowing the facets to create a joint between each vertebra. The pedicles have notches which form an opening, allowing the spinal nerves an exit point from the cord.

5.1   CERVICAL SPINE

The cervical spine is made up of the first seven vertebrae and functions to provide mobility and stability to the head, while connecting it to the relatively immobile thoracic spine. It has a natural lordotic curve and the smallest movable vertebrae. C3–6 have common features but C1–2 and C7 have their own special features. The first two vertebral bodies are quite different from the rest of the cervical spine. The atlas, or C1 (**Fig 1.1-6**), articulates superiorly with the occiput and inferiorly with the axis or C2 (**Fig 1.1-7**).

The atlas has no body or spinous process but develops as a ring of bone with anterior and posterior arches that connect two lateral masses. During development of the atlas, what should

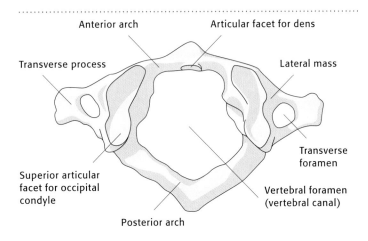

Fig 1.1-6
Atlas or C1.

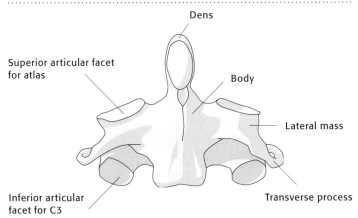

Fig 1.1-7
Axis or C2.

be the body becomes naturally fused to the axis forming the dens or odontoid peg and therefore is presented as the body of the axis. This is approximately 1.5 cm in length and seen as a tooth-like structure which acts as a central point to allow rotation for the atlas.

The joints or facets are seated on top of each other to form the lateral mass. This is a building block of bone, which supports the occiput. What is also unique at this level of the spine is that there is no disc between C1 and C2.

The remaining cervical vertebrae, C3–7, are similar to each other but are very different from C1 and C2. They each have a vertebral body, which is concave on its superior surface and convex on its inferior surface. The spinous processes of C3–5 are usually bifid, in comparison to the spinous processes of C6 and C7, which are usually tapered (**Fig 1.1-8, Fig 1.1-9**).

5.2   THORACIC SPINE

The thoracic section consists of twelve vertebrae, T1–12. It has a natural kyphotic curve and is rigid due to the fact that it articulates with the twelve pairs of ribs (**Fig 1.1-10**). As we travel down the thoracic spine, the vertebrae enlarge in size. The apex is usually found at T7/8, and it is at this level that the discs have a major role in influencing the curve.

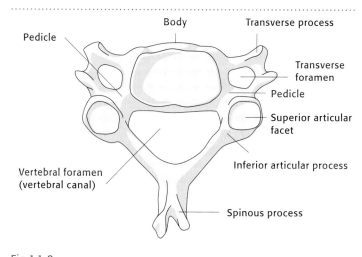

Fig 1.1-8
Cervical vertebra.

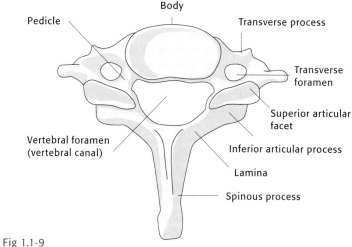

Fig 1.1-9
7th cervical vertebra.

Like the cervical spine, the thoracic spine also has distinct identifying features, and will be addressed where differences can be seen.

Marked differences evolve in the thoracic spine. Near the root of the pedicle there are two demi-facets, the superior costal facet and the inferior costal facet. Both are covered by cartilage and form an oval surface to accommodate the heads of the corresponding ribs. There is also a small costal facet on the transverse process which connects to the tubercle of the rib.

T1 has a single articular costal facet for the head of the 1st rib. The lower facets are much smaller so as to house the upper half of the 2nd rib.

T6 demonstrates how the spinous process is longer and extends downwards in the thoracic spine (**Fig 1.1-11, Fig 1.1-12**).

T9, while having the same characteristics as T1–8, fails to form a connection with the 10th rib, so the inferior costal facets on the body are not present.

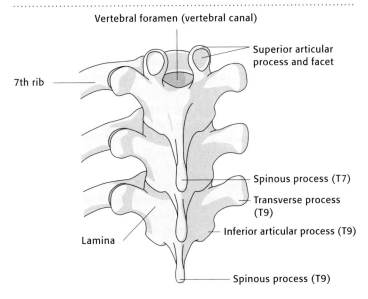

Fig 1.1-10
The posterior view of the thoracic spine.

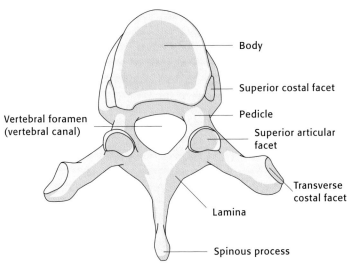

Fig 1.1-11
The superior view of T6.

T10 only articulates with the 10th rib and has no connection to the 11th rib, so in this situation only the superior costal facet on the body is present. The transverse process facet at this level may not be present.

T11 articulates only with the 11th rib at the head and protrudes more to the pedicles. The transverse processes are small, with no evidence of the facets for the tubercle connection.

T12 articulates only with the 12th rib below the upper body and encroaches onto the pedicle; it is at this level that similarities are found with the lumbar spine (**Fig 1.1-13**).

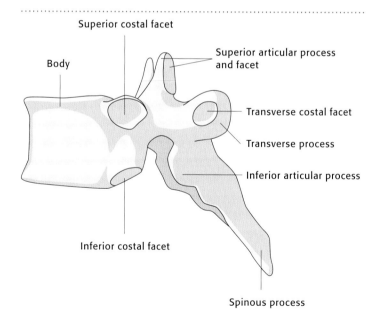

Superior costal facet

Body

Superior articular process and facet

Transverse costal facet

Transverse process

Inferior articular process

Inferior costal facet

Spinous process

Fig 1.1-12
The lateral view of T6.

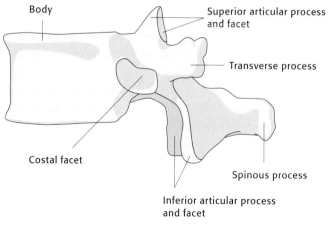

Body

Superior articular process and facet

Transverse process

Costal facet

Spinous process

Inferior articular process and facet

Fig 1.1-13
The lateral view of T12.

5.3   LUMBAR SPINE

The lumbar section consists of five vertebrae, L1–5. It has a natural lordotic curve and is much larger in size. The spinous process is thicker and the pedicles are shorter, but the body is much larger, fairly flat, and broad in shape. The lumbar spine is more mobile than the rigid thoracic spine but lacks the flexibility of the cervical spine. It is at this level that most weight is centered, and thus it sustains the greatest stresses. The distinguishing landmarks at this level are very large transverse processes that connect to all the lateral surfaces of the pedicles and also encroach onto the side of the vertebral body (**Fig 1.1-14**).

5.4   SACRUM

The sacrum section appears triangular and consists of five fused vertebrae (**Fig 1.1-15**). The purpose of this area of the spine is to transmit body weight to the hips. It articulates with the pelvis via the sacroiliac joints. The sacrum is angulated; the base presents downwards and forwards and has an important outcome on the mechanics of the spine and pelvis.

The posterior surface has crests over the fused spinous, articular, and transverse processes. This is known as the median sacral crest. The first vertebra is known as the sacral promon-

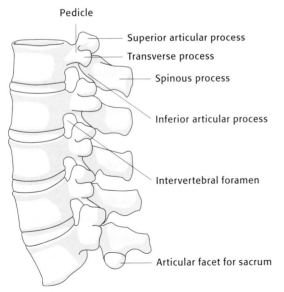

Fig 1.1-14
Lateral view of the lumbar vertebrae.

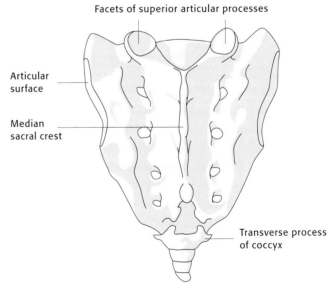

Fig 1.1-15
The posterior surface of the sacrum and coccyx.

tory because of the high profile ridge. The sacral ala is the flat broad area where the S1 articulates with the ilium of the pelvis.

5.5   COCCYX

The coccyx section is a small triangular-shaped bone which consists of four undeveloped vertebrae fused together and is the most caudal section of the spinal column; however, the number of vertebrae present can vary from five to three (**Fig 1.1-15**).

5.6   RIBS

The ribs usually consist of twelve pairs but in some cases cervical and lumbar ribs have developed, and it has been documented that cervical ribs have been found as high as C4. The direction in which the rib forms can vary. They consist of a shaft with an anterior and posterior end and are marked along the stem by a costal groove. At the posterior end it consists of a head, neck, and the articular and nonarticular section of the tubercle (**Fig 1.1-16a–b**).

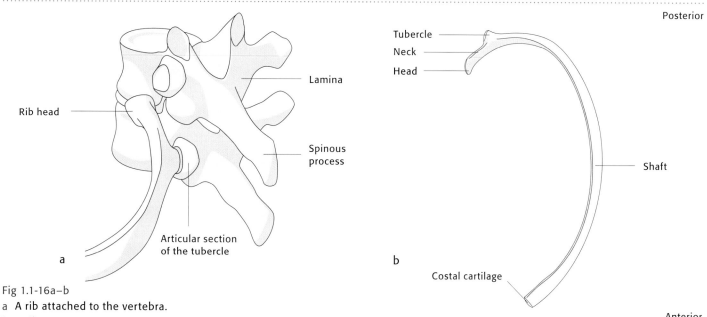

Fig 1.1-16a–b
a   A rib attached to the vertebra.
b   A rib.

They are denoted into three sections: true, false, and floating.

- R1–6 are true.
- R7–10 are false.
- R11–12 are floating.

True ribs are linked by means of costal cartilages and the sternum, which applies to R1–6.

False ribs are where the costal cartilages are joined to the rib above, which applies to R7–10.

Floating ribs are not linked to the sternum, which applies to R11–12. Just like the vertebrae, they also have distinguishing features.

R1: This may be the smallest rib; however, it boasts the largest curve. The head has only one facet used to articulate with the T1 vertebra and an oval facet for articulation with the transverse process. If there is any variation of angulations on this it could have an effect on the brachial plexus and subclavian vessels causing traction or entrapment.

R2: This is twice the size in length than R1 but has a similar curve.

R10: This has a single facet on the head, which will articulate with both the vertebral body and also the T9/10 disc.

R11–12: These ribs do not have necks or tubercles; however, they do have a large single articulating facet. R11 has a slight angle, whereas on rib R12 the angle is absent and the rib is much shorter.

6   INTERVERTEBRAL JOINT

A simple joint of the spine would be two vertebral bodies united at their smooth ends, which would not only allow a gliding movement for each pair, but also be strong enough for weight bearing. However, if the vertebral column is to succeed in its anatomical duty, with regard to flexion and extension or lateral bending, the surface of the joints would require modification to accommodate these movements (**Fig 1.1-17a–b**). This modification would compromise the stability of the joint and also the weight-bearing role required so therefore would be unsuitable for this section of the human skeleton. Nature created the intervertebral disc with which to separate the two bodies and allow the upper vertebra to tilt without contact on its lower partner.

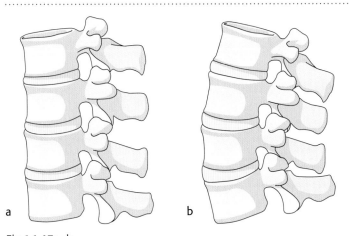

Fig 1.1-17a–b
a Flexion.
b Extension.

6.1   VERTEBRAL END PLATES

In the young the vertebral end plates consist of hyaline carti-lage and fibrocartilage, in the mature disc they are virtually all fibrocartilage.

During growth they are responsible for the depth of the verte-bral body and are considered part of the disc. They measure 0.6–1 mm thick. The two end plates of each disc cover the nu-cleus pulposus completely but fail to cover the annulus fibro-sus entirely (**Fig 1.1-18**). These end plates have two other im-portant roles:

- Nutrition of the disc: the end plates form a porous barrier allowing water and nutrients to pass between the nucleus pulposus and cancellous bone of the vertebral body.

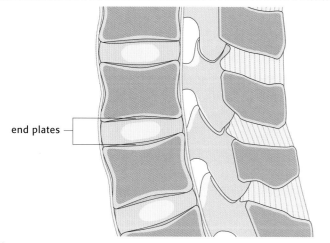

Fig 1.1-18
An end plate of the body.

- The mechanical role is to prevent the nucleus bulging into the vertebral body.

The end plates are considered to be the weakest part of the disc.

6.2   INTERVERTEBRAL DISC

There are three biomechanical goals the disc must be able to achieve:

- The strength to sustain the weight distribution load from one vertebra to the other.
- The flexibility to allow forward movement in flexion, backward movement in extension, and limited movement from side to side laterally, plus rotation.
- The strength to prevent injury during any movement.

The cushion-like structure acts as a shock absorber during ac-tivity. The discs are thickest at the cervical and lumbar regions, which constitute approximately one-quarter of the entire height of the spine. The overall body height decreases between 15–20 mm during the day, this is due to loss of disc height and prolonged loading. The loss of height is recuperated during the night.

The upper four thoracic discs decrease in thickness, then in-crease down to the 10th level. The lumbosacral joint is the largest and most noticeably dense interiorly.

The disc is made up of two components: a tough ring called annulus fibrosus, and the nucleus pulposus which is made up of a semi-fluid gel. The nucleus provides elasticity and compressibility while the annulus fibrosus contains and limits the expansion of the nucleus (**Fig 1.1-19**).

• Nucleus pulposus
  This consists of finer (type ll) collagen fibers arranged in a loose mesh, and semi-fluid proteoglycan gel with a consistency similar to toothpaste, which makes up 40–60% of the disc. The hydrophitic nature of the proteoglycan gel means that the nucleus can become deformed when under pressure without loss of volume. This is an advantage in accommodating movement and the transfer of compressive load from one vertebra to the next—it is able to change shape when under pressure from any direction, therefore transmitting the applied pressure in all directions.

• Annulus fibrosus
  This consists of concentric laminal layers of (type l) collagen fibers. Attached to the annulus are the anterior and posterior longitudinal ligaments.

The disc is avascular after the age of 10 years and relies on the diffusion of nutrients such as oxygen, glucose, and sulfate.

This is achieved in two ways:

• Blood vessels around the annulus fibrosus.
• Capillary plexuses under the end plates.

The nucleus accepts almost all its nutrition via the end-plate pathway.

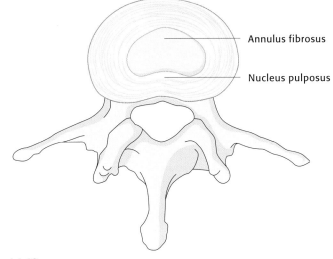

Annulus fibrosus

Nucleus pulposus

Fig 1.1-19
Disc.

7   LIGAMENTS

To enable the bones of the spine to maintain stability in the upright position, the ligaments and muscles are there as a support mechanism. A ligament is described as a connecting tissue from one bone to another (**Fig 1.1-20**). Bone injury to the spine with ligamentous damage can determine the surgical plan. When reducing the bone injury, the ligament can aid restoration of the bone anatomy back to its anatomical position to help maintain stability.

There are six important ligaments associated with the spine:

- Anterior longitudinal ligament
  This is a strong band which extends from the anterior aspect at the base of the occipital bone, via the atlas and down the anterior surface of each vertebra and disc to the sacrum. It is approximately 20 mm wide and is a collagen ligament made up of three layers. Its role is to prevent anterior separation of each vertebral body when in extension and flexion.

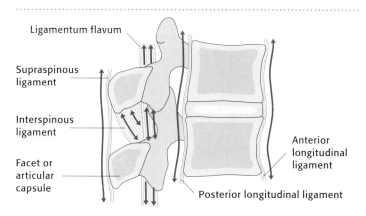

Fig 1.1-20 Lateral view of ligaments in the lumbar spine.

Ligamentum flavum

Supraspinous ligament

Interspinous ligament

Facet or articular capsule

Anterior longitudinal ligament

Posterior longitudinal ligament

- Posterior longitudinal ligament
  This is also a strong band, but lying posterior to the bodies and discs, which extends from the posterior aspect at the base of the occipital bone, via the dens or odontoid peg and down the posterior surface of each vertebra and disc to the coccyx. Unlike the anterior ligaments, it is broader over the discs and narrow over the bodies.

- Supraspinous ligament
  This is a fibrous cord that attaches at the tips of each spinous process. This ligament ceases between L4 and L5. Below this, fibers from the thoracolumbar facia take over the role providing strength and sagittal movement at the lumbosacral junction.

- Interspinous ligament
  This connects adjacent spinous processes. Their appearance is thin at the thoracic section and starts where the spine overlaps. This ligament differs from others in its lack of continuity, and by its presentation as a series of short ligaments.

- Ligamentum flavum
  These ligaments are short and thick and protect the disc by limiting movement. They are also known as the yellow ligament due to their distinctive color. The elasticity of these ligaments is greater than the other ligaments and represents the most elastic tissue in the human body.

- Facet or articular capsule
  These surround the zygapophyeal joint found at the superior and inferior articular processes. They are thin and loose, which allows movement in the sagittal plane.

8   MUSCLES

Muscles create a cover of soft tissues, which permits movement and stability of the spinal column. As a group they are known as the paraspinal muscles. Their role is to stabilize all the bones, influence posture, and extend, flex, and rotate the spinal column. Muscles work together as a team, but each one has a part to play.

Muscle fibers of the spine vary in length. Short muscle fibers lie the deepest, while long muscle fibers may be described as a system of guy ropes.

8.1   ANTERIOR MUSCLES

The muscles associated with flexion (**Fig 1.1-21**) include:

- Longus capitis, which extends from the lateral masses to the foramen magnum.
- Longus colli, which extends from the atlas to T3.
- Psoas major, which lies in the lumbar region and extends into the hip.
- Psoas minor, which lies on the surface of the psoas major from T12–L1. The psoas minor is found in only two out of every three patients.

8.2   POSTERIOR MUSCLES

The posterior consists of a collection of mainly longitudinal extensor muscles, which run the whole length of the vertebral column from the skull to the sacrum. They form a projection on either side of the midline of the back, which is predominantly noticeable in the lumbar region.

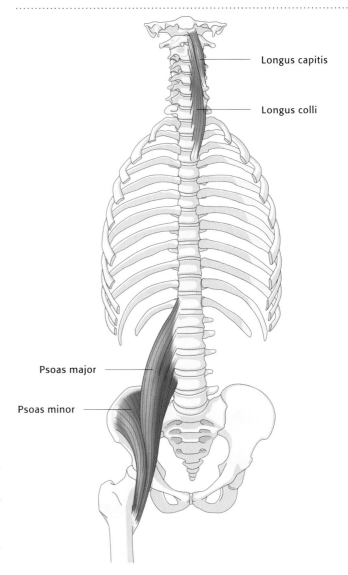

Fig 1.1-21
Anterior muscles.

There are three layers of posterior muscles:

- deep
- intermediate
- superficial

The deep layers are the interspinales and intertransversales muscles, which connect the spinous and transverse processes to each other. These muscles are small and considered unimportant.

The intermediate layers are the transversospinalis muscles, which extend from the transverse processes to the spine (**Fig 1.1-22**). This layer includes the following groups:

- multifidus
- semispinalis thoracis
- semispinalis cervicis
- semispinalis capitis

All have a part to play in rotation, each in different regions pertaining to the bone anatomy of the spine.

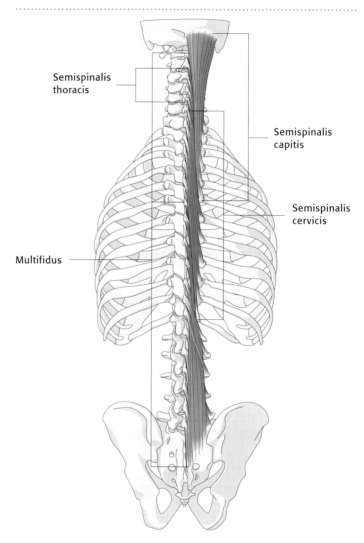

Semispinalis thoracis

Semispinalis capitis

Semispinalis cervicis

Multifidus

Fig 1.1-22
Posterior: intermediate muscles.

The superficial layers are the erector spinae, which forms the most powerful muscle group associated with the spine (**Fig 1.1-23**). This group consists of the following:

- iliocostalis
- longissimus: capitis, cervicis, and thoracis
- spinalis cervicis
- spinalis thoracis

There are further external muscles controlling movement of the body around the spine and include such muscles as:

- serratus posterior superior
- rhomboid minor
- trapezius
- rhomboid major
- latissimus dorsi
- serratus posterior inferior

The whole mass of back muscles consists in large numbers alongside tendon bundles. Back pain can be due to stretching and tearing between muscles, tendons, and bone, and this can occur at multiple sites in the back, spinal cord, and nerves.

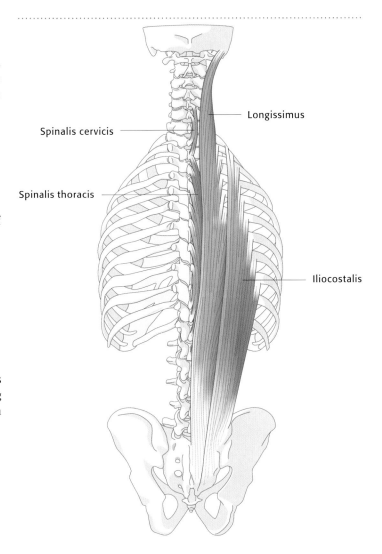

Fig 1.1-23
Posterior: superficial muscles.

9   SPINAL CORD AND NERVES

Knowledge of the neurology pertaining to the spine is essential for treatment and medical management of spine disorders. It also allows for an understanding of the clinical symptoms of degenerative disease.

9.1   SPINAL CORD

The cord is housed within the vertebral foramen and is therefore protected by bone. It is seen as a solitary integrated organ, cylindrical in shape. It extends from the foramen magnum, the entry point at the base of the skull. It connects to the medulla oblongata at this point. The cord ends at around the L1/L2 disc (**Fig 1.1-24**).

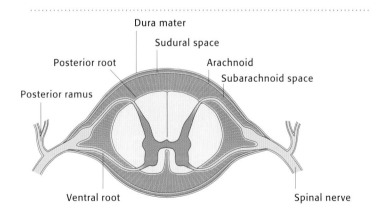

Fig 1.1-24
Membranes of the cord.

Below this level it divides at the conus medullaris, seen as a bundle of filaments. This bundle consists of the lumbar and sacral nerve roots. They resemble a horse's tail and are called the cauda equina. At the most distal point it is attached to the coccyx by the filum terminable. This is a nonnervous structure, which is an extension of the pia mater and encased by the dura mater (both membranes).

There are three membranes surrounding the cord. As a group they are known as meninges:

- Dura mater: external loose sheath, which does not adhere to the cord.
- Arachnoid: thin delicate layer between the dura mater and pia mater.
- Pia mater: innermost layer which adheres to the cord.

Between the dura mater and the arachnoid is an area called the subdural space, containing serous fluid. Between the pia mater and the arachnoid is an area called the subarachnoid space, which contains a serous secretion known as cerebrospinal fluid (CSF). This fluid supports the meninges and disperses forces acting through them.

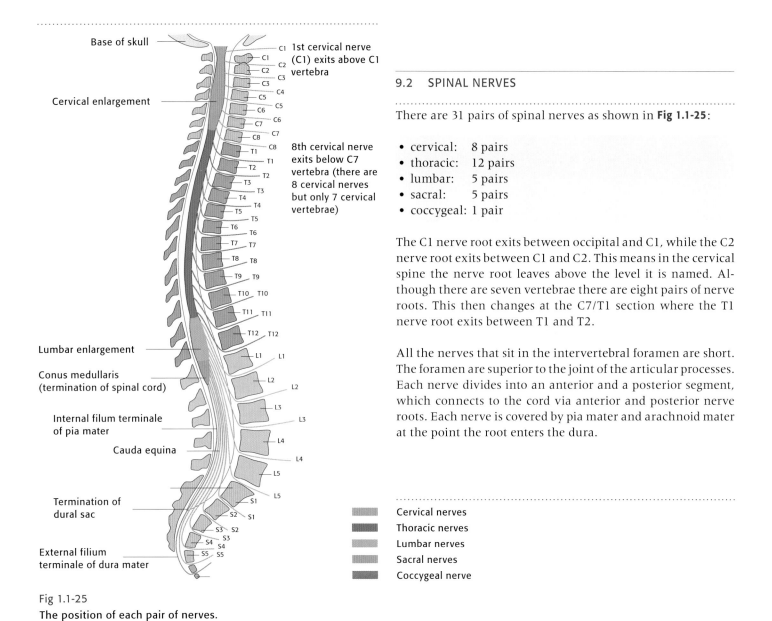

Base of skull

C1   1st cervical nerve
C1   (C1) exits above C1
C2   vertebra
C2
C3
C3
Cervical enlargement
C4
C5
C5
C6
C6
C7
C7
C8
C8   8th cervical nerve
T1   exits below C7
T1   vertebra (there are
T2   8 cervical nerves
T2   but only 7 cervical
T3   vertebrae)
T3
T4
T4
T5
T5
T6
T6
T7
T7
T8
T8
T9
T9
T10   T10
T11   T11
T12   T12

Lumbar enlargement
L1   L1

Conus medullaris
(termination of spinal cord)
L2   L2

L3
L3
Internal filum terminale
of pia mater
L4

Cauda equina
L4

L5
L5
Termination of
dural sac
S1
S2   S1
S3   S2
External filium
S4   S3
terminale of dura mater
S5   S4
S5   S5

Fig 1.1-25
The position of each pair of nerves.

Cervical nerves
Thoracic nerves
Lumbar nerves
Sacral nerves
Coccygeal nerve

9.2   SPINAL NERVES

There are 31 pairs of spinal nerves as shown in **Fig 1.1-25**:

- cervical: 8 pairs
- thoracic: 12 pairs
- lumbar: 5 pairs
- sacral: 5 pairs
- coccygeal: 1 pair

The C1 nerve root exits between occipital and C1, while the C2 nerve root exits between C1 and C2. This means in the cervical spine the nerve root leaves above the level it is named. Although there are seven vertebrae there are eight pairs of nerve roots. This then changes at the C7/T1 section where the T1 nerve root exits between T1 and T2.

All the nerves that sit in the intervertebral foramen are short. The foramen are superior to the joint of the articular processes. Each nerve divides into an anterior and a posterior segment, which connects to the cord via anterior and posterior nerve roots. Each nerve is covered by pia mater and arachnoid mater at the point the root enters the dura.

The anterior nerve root acts as a motor nerve, the posterior nerve root provides sensory information, and a posterior and anterior root attaches these to the cord.

The plexus network is an additional branch of the nerves. They communicate with neighboring nerves in which to innervate certain areas of the human body.

Through continuous division and reformation, the plexus is formed. The plexi are divided into four main divisions:

- Cervical plexus: due to the anterior division of the upper four cervical nerves.
- Brachial plexus: due to the merger of the anterior division of the lower four cervical nerves and the first thoracic nerve.
- Lumbar plexus: due to the anterior division of the upper four lumbar nerves and the twelfth thoracic nerve.
- Sacral plexus: due to the lumbosacral cord, anterior division of upper three sacral nerves, and a section of the fourth sacral nerve.

Through this interchange of fibers, all the nerves exiting the plexus have an improved connection with the cord, perhaps more so than if it had taken a direct route.

10   DERMATOMES

The sensory component of each spinal nerve distributes to a segmental part of the skin called a dermatome. The pattern of skin distribution generally follows the segmental distribution of underlying muscle innervations. Testing the sensation on the skin as well as testing motor power is useful in determining the presence of a nerve, spinal tract, or spinal cord lesion (**Fig 1.1-26a–b**).

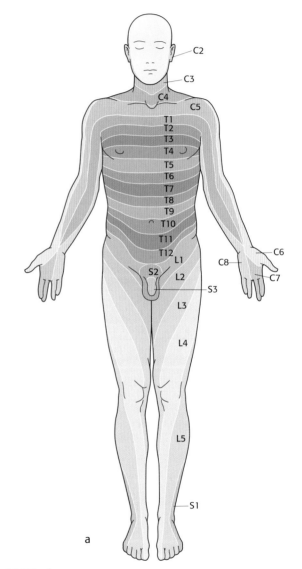

Fig 1.1-26a–b
Dermatome map.

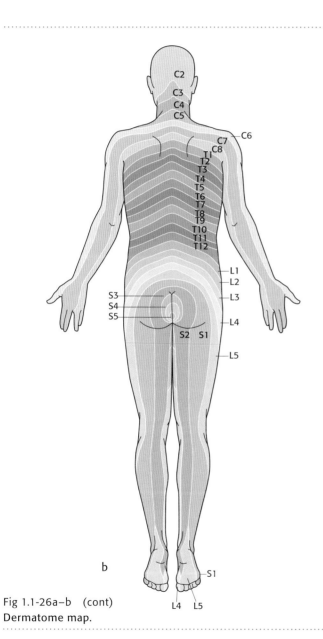

11 SUGGESTIONS FOR FURTHER READING

Bogduk N (2003) *Clinical Anatomy of the Lumbar Spine and Sacrum.* 3rd ed. London: Churchill Livingstone.
Clancy J, McVicar A, Williams M (2000) The musculo-skeletal system. The spine. *Br J Perioper Nurs;* 10(11):568–576.
McMinn RM (1994) *Last's Anatomy—regional and applied.* 9th ed. London: Churchill Livingstone.
Oliver J, Middleditch A (1991) *Functional Anatomy of the Spine.* 1st ed. Oxford: Butterworth-Heinemann Ltd.
Williams PL, Warwick R (1980) *Gray's Anatomy.* 36th ed. London: Churchill Livingstone.

Fig 1.1-26a–b (cont)
Dermatome map.

1.2   IMAGING OF THE SPINE

1   INTRODUCTION

The outcome of surgical management for spinal disorders is dependent on appropriate patient selection. This is achieved by a combination of clinical assessment, namely an accurate history and thorough physical examination, aided by appropriate imaging of the spine.

Imaging aids in the diagnosis of spinal pathology, the site and extent of the disease, and in quantification of deformity. It is essential in preoperative planning. This chapter will outline the imaging modalities utilized in spinal patients and the use of mobile radiography (fluoroscopy) in the operating room.

Diagnostic imaging studies used in spinal disorders include plain radiography, magnetic resonance imaging (MRI), computed tomography (CT), and bone scanning.

2   PLAIN RADIOGRAPHY

X-rays were discovered by Wilhelm Röntgen in 1895 and were so named due to the uncertainty of their nature. They are occasionally referred to as Röntgen's rays and the picture obtained from exposing film to x-rays is a Röntgenogram or radiograph—but is more commonly and incorrectly referred to as an x-ray.

X-rays are electromagnetic radiation waves with a very short wavelength which are powerful enough to penetrate most substances other than the heavy metals such as gold or lead. X-rays are generated within a low-pressure chamber present within an x-ray machine by firing a stream of electrons at a metal target. An electron stream is produced by passing an extremely high potential difference (voltage) between a positive tungsten coiled element (cathode), and a negatively charged rotating tungsten alloy disc (anode). As the electrons slow down on hitting this metal target, electromagnetic radiation waves (x-rays) are produced. The cathode heats to 2,500°C and the anode spins at up to 10,000 rotations per minute to prevent overheating—this is the whirring noise heard when an x-ray is taken.

The x-rays produced by this method are directed towards the subject and are absorbed to a differing degree by tissues, dependent on their composition and densities. An x-ray plate behind the subject containing a phosphor/activator compound can subsequently be developed in a dark room, and reflects the x-ray radiation passing through the subject. Tissues that are less dense (ie, air-filled lung tissue) are dark on a plain x-ray (radiopaque); dense structures such as bone appear white (radiodense).

In the spine, plain x-rays are a base-line investigation required in most clinical scenarios. There are several different views of the spine; the indications for each are outlined in **Table 1.2-1**.

Indication	Views	Main features
Cervical trauma	Lateral including C1–T7 (**Fig 1.2-1**) Swimmers view Anteroposterior (AP) Open mouth peg view (**Fig 1.2-2**) ± right and left 45° oblique Lateral view with traction of both arms (upper limbs)	Soft-tissue swelling Bony alignment Fracture
Thoracolumbar trauma	AP Lateral Standing lateral (if clinically indicated)	Bony alignment Spinous process rotation Interspinous widening Interpedicular widening Kyphotic deformity/wedging
Low back pain	AP (**Fig 1.2-3, 1.2-4**) Lateral ± coned view of lumbosacral junction	Loss of disc space height Syndesmophytes (osteophytes) Degenerative spondylolisthesis

Table 1.2-1
Plain radiographic spinal views.

Indication	Views	Main features
Scoliosis	Whole spine standing lateral Whole spine standing AP (**Fig 1.2-5**) Fulcrum bending films	Sagittal and coronal alignment Cobb angle of curves Vertebral body rotation Congenital abnormalities Flexibility on bending
Kyphosis	Whole spine AP standing Whole spine lateral standing Hyperextension films	Sagittal balance Cobb angle of kyphosis Flexibility on hyperextension
Tumor	Chest AP Lateral	Metastatic/primary lung lesion Pedicle destruction Vertebral body collapse
Spondylolisthesis	AP Coned lateral of the lumbosacral junction Ferguson view	Degree of slip of one vertebra on another Pars defect
Infection	AP Lateral	Disc space reduction or increase Vertebral body collapse Loss of psoas shadow Gas

Table 1.2-1 (cont)
Plain radiographic spinal views.

During surgery, the preoperative x-rays should be placed on the operating room viewing box as they are referred to throughout surgery for both confirmation of bony anatomy and for the profile of the spine for the accurate placement of implants. It is normal practice for the AP x-ray to be oriented as though the patient is being viewed from behind—spine surgeons view the spine in this orientation while examining patients and the majority of spine surgery is through a posterior approach.

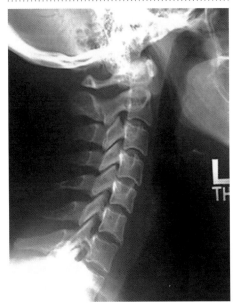

Fig 1.2-1
Normal lateral cervical spine x-ray.

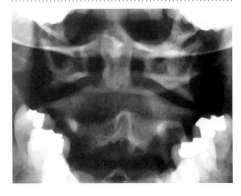

Fig 1.2-2
Open mouth view to show normal anatomical relationship of the upper cervical spine or C0–2.

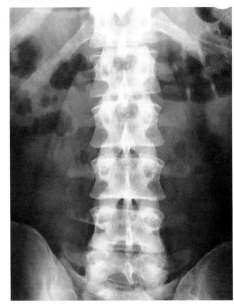

Fig 1.2-3
Plain AP x-ray of the lumbar spine.

Intraoperative plain x-rays are taken by most surgeons to identify or confirm the anatomical level at which they are operating, as direct visualization of anatomy can be misleading. They are thought, by some, to be essential for documentation of the surgery being carried out at the correct level and, therefore, protective from a medicolegal point of view.

Limited surgical exposure techniques require confirmation of level using intraoperative imaging. The x-ray plate is covered with a sterile drape in a holder, placed parallel to the spine and perpendicular to the x-ray beam (**Fig 1.2-6**). A qualified radiographer operates a mobile x-ray machine after appropriate precautions have been taken for staff and patient safety.

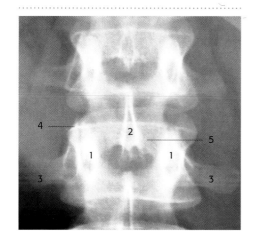

Fig 1.2-4
AP x-ray of the lumbar spine.
1   Pedicle
2   Spinous process
3   Transverse process
4   Facet joint
5   Lamina

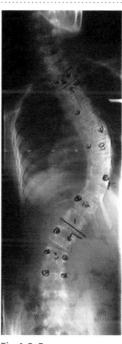

Fig 1.2-5
Standing AP scoliogram.

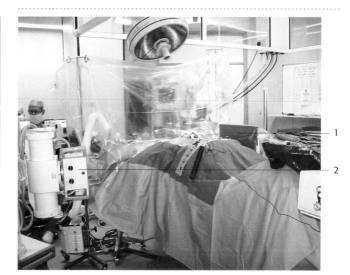

Fig 1.2-6
Operating room set-up for intraoperative x-ray.
1   Sterile covered plate
2   X-ray machine

3   IMAGE INTENSIFIER AND FLUOROSCOPY

A fluoroscope uses an x-ray tube and a fluoroscopic screen (**Fig 1.2-7**) to generate immediate imaging of a subject viewed on a monitor. Varying exposure time can create a real time x-ray movie, and a brief exposure time results in a snapshot picture. The image is inverted as compared to a conventional x-ray, with radiodense structures appearing dark and radiopaque structures appearing light. The use of an image intensifier or C-arm is commonplace in spine surgery and can have several uses including:

- localization of operative level,
- placement of needle in injection techniques,
- reduction of fracture confirmation,
- insertion of pedicle screws.

The commonest use of the image intensifier is for:

- percutaneous needle placement for discography,
- nerve root blocks,
- facet joint injections (**Fig 1.2-8**),
- foraminal epidurals.

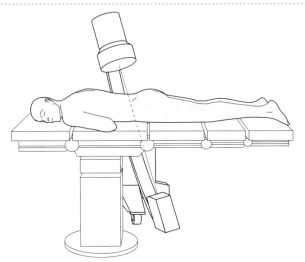

Fig 1.2-7
Image intensifier positioned for facet joint injections.

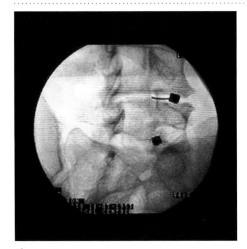

Fig 1.2-8
Inverted image on monitor of image intensifier during facet joint injections.

4   MAGNETIC RESONANCE IMAGING

The advantage of magnetic resonance imaging (MRI) in the spine is its visualization of soft tissues. Although providing invaluable information on spinal pathology, MRI complements but does not replace a sound history and full clinical examination.

Images are created from a signal received in a coil surrounding the patient as elements with odd numbers of protons (hydrogen) return to align with a strong magnetic field after being exposed to a brief radio frequency signal.

The magnet of an MRI scanner has a magnetic field of some 30,000 times that of the earth. The time after "relaxation" of the radio frequency burst at which the signal received in the coil is captured determines the "weighting" of the produced image. Commonly produced images are referred to as T1 (fast) or T2 (slow) weighted imaging. As a rule of thumb, fat appears as high signal (white) in T1-weighted images and water as low signal (dark); in T2-weighted images water appears as high signal (white) and fat as low signal (dark). With particular reference to the spine, cerebrospinal fluid is white on T2 images and can be clearly seen surrounding the spinal cord and the cauda equina.

Intervertebral discs in the nondegenerate spine appear light due to water content within them—as the degenerative process sets in, the hydration of the disc reduces and so leaves the disc appearing dark (**Table 1.2-2**). The term black disc disease has been attributed to this process. Bright signal changes within the end plates of vertebral bodies adjacent to a degenerative disc are a normal reaction and are referred to as Modic changes [1]. Changes within end plates around a nondegenerative high intensity disc may represent an infective process within the disc (**Fig 1.2-9a–b**).

	T1	T2
Fat including bone marrow	White	Grey
Water	Grey	White
Trauma/hemorrhage	Grey	White
Tumor	Grey	White
Inflammation	Grey	White
Infection	Grey	White
Scarring and ligaments	Grey/black	Grey/black
Calcium/cortical bone	Black	Black
Muscle	Grey	Grey
Normal intervertebral disc: peripheral	Black	Grey
Normal intervertebral disc: central	Grey	White
Degenerative disc	Black	Black

Table 1.2-2
Examples of MRI signal intensity.

MRI images are obtained in three planes: frontal, axial, and sagittal—the latter two are more common in the assessment of spinal pathology. T1 images are generally better at picking up pathology such as tumors, whereas T2 images show anatomy clearly. MRI imaging of structures in the vicinity of implants may appear blurred, making interpretation difficult. Titanium implants are preferred if further MRI is expected (ie, following the stabilization of tumor) as it gives significantly less artifact than stainless steel.

Due to the strength of the magnet within the MRI scanner, patients who have:

- pacemakers,
- intracerebral aneurysm clips,
- internal hearing aids,
- or metallic orbital foreign bodies

are restricted from being scanned.

For these patients alternative methods of imaging must be found, for example CT myelography (CT after intrathecal contrast injection).

An MRI scan of the whole spine requires the patient to be still inside a close, narrow, and noisy tunnel for 20 minutes—approximately 15% of patients cannot tolerate this procedure due to claustrophobia and may require sedation. Otherwise, an open MRI can be used where available. MRI has the added advantage of being radiation free.

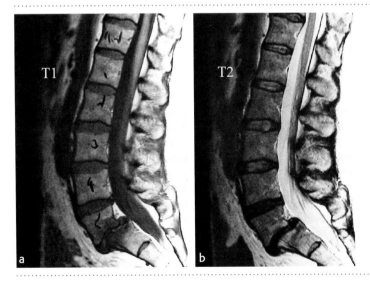

Fig 1.2-9a–b
T1 and T2 images of degenerative spondylolisthesis. Note the dark signal within the L4/5 and L5/S1 discs showing degeneration and the slip of L5 on S1.

5   COMPUTED TOMOGRAPHY

Tomography is the production of a radiograph focused in a single plane with removal of the outline of structures in other planes. Computed tomography (CT) uses a computer for image reconstruction following the acquisition of multiple x-ray images from different angles. In practice this is achieved by rotating an x-ray source around the subject opposite a static ring-shaped detector.

CT produces axially sliced images through the body and it is possible to reformat these images in any required plane. Striking 3-D images add to the understanding of complex congenital deformity (**Fig 1.2-10**). The strength of CT in the spine is its ability to define the anatomy of bone, making it ideal for the

assessment of spinal fractures and the preoperative planning of screw placement, particularly in proximal cervical spine fixation where pedicle width and foramina position is paramount. It is less useful in visualization of soft tissues in comparison to MRI.

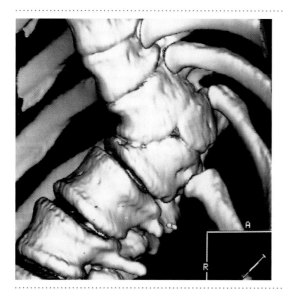

Fig 1.2-10
3-D reconstruction of hemivertebrae.

6   BONE SCAN

A bone scan involves the intravenous injection of a radiolabelled diphosphonate technetium-99, which combines with calcium in areas of bone with an increased cell turnover, mineralization, or blood flow. Increased bone turnover is seen in healing bone, growth plates of immature bones and reactive bone change to degenerative joint disease. Increased blood flow occurs in fractures, inflammation, infection, and tumors.

Practically, the patient is scanned by a gamma camera three times (triple phase bone scan)—just after injection (flow phase), at 10 minutes (blood pool phase), and at 4 hours (delayed phase). Bone scans are helpful in the exclusion of serious pathology in the patient with back pain. They are very sensitive to bone tumors (primary or secondary) and infection; analysis of the three phases can often differentiate between these. The axial skeleton is a common site of metastatic bone deposits from lung, breast, and prostate tumors and patients commonly present to the spine surgeon with neurological deficit, instability, or pain. It is vital to know whether a patient has solitary or multiple metastatic bone lesions as this may influence management.

7   SAFETY AND PROTECTION

The current dose limit from x-rays is 20 millisieverts (mSv) per year for employees. Exposure to high-dose radiation has the potential risk of a detrimental health effect, malignancy and genetic aberration in the unborn. Studies have shown operating room personnel (ORP) should remain a minimum of 46–70 cm away from the x-ray beam to receive only low-dose radiation and a distance of greater than 90 cm is considered an extremely low exposure risk [2]. Further recent evidence suggests that at a distance greater than 2 m from the x-ray beam, the radiation dose received is minimal [3]. Although in general the radiation dose received in the operating room has consistently been recorded as low, the effects of long-term exposure to this low dose have not been accurately determined, therefore making it common sense to avoid unnecessary exposure.

Due to the nature of image intensifier use in spine surgery requiring multiple x-ray exposures, ORP should wear a lead-protective gown (0.25 mm thick) when working in a controlled area (OR) as outlined in local rules under the Ionizing Radiations Regulations 199917 (IRR99). Both the surgeon performing the procedure and the scrub personnel should wear a thyroid shield, as there is an increased risk of thyroid cancer after radiation exposure. Guidelines from the National Radiation Protection Board suggest that ionizing radiation from man-made and natural sources may place an additional risk of fatal cancer in the region of 1% over a lifetime as compared to a 25% overall lifetime risk of cancer from all causes. Medical radiation may account for as high as 14% of the overall life-time radiation dose.

The doses involved in spinal imaging can be significant. A single lateral view of the whole spine requires a dose of 2 mSv and is the equivalent of 200 chest x-rays or 12 months background radiation. A bone scan is 4 mSv and a CT scan of the abdomen and chest 18 mSv—the equivalent of 2.3 and 8 years background radiation respectively. It is estimated that a helical CT scan of the abdomen in a young girl results in a risk of fatal cancer of 1 in 1,000 attributable to that scan [4]. It is with this in mind the use of imaging involving radiation exposure be limited and justified on clinical grounds.

8   BIBLIOGRAPHY

1. **Modic MT, Steinberg PM, Ross JS, et al** (1988) Degenerative disc disease: assessment of changes in vertebral body marrow with MR imaging. *Radiology;* 166:193–199.

2. **Mehlman CT, DiPasquale TG** (1997) Radiation exposure to the orthopedic surgical team during fluoroscopy: "how far away is far enough?". *J Orthop Trauma;* 11(6):392–398.

3. **Alonso JA, Shaw DL, Maxwell A, et al** (2001) Scattered radiation during fixation of hip fractures. Is distance alone enough protection? *J Bone Joint Surg Br;* 83(6):815–818.

4. **Brenner D, Elliston C, Hall E, et al** (2001) Estimated risks of radiation-induced fatal cancer from pediatric CT. *AJR Am J Roentgenol;* 176(2):289–296.

1.3   SPINAL CORD MONITORING

1   INTRODUCTION

Various techniques for intraoperative monitoring of spinal cord function have been developed over the past 25 years. Severe neurological complications may occur following surgical correction of a spinal deformity and traditionally the wake-up test was used. The use of intraoperative spinal cord monitoring was introduced in an attempt to replace the wake-up test. However, the wake-up test is still used occasionally today, and is considered by some to be the gold standard.

Each method of monitoring does have disadvantages. Performed properly, the wake-up test reveals the status of the patient's motor function at the time as which it is performed. The primary disadvantage of this test is that the patient's motor function can only be ascertained at that particular moment in time, unless repeated wake-up tests are performed during the procedure.

Intraoperative spinal cord monitoring identifies any changes in spinal cord function resulting from vascular compromise, trauma during fitting of the instrumentation, or direct mechanical stretching of the cord.

These techniques permit early recognition of any changes in spinal cord function, and therefore allow appropriate measures to be taken immediately, thus preventing irreversible damage occurring.

The use of spinal cord monitoring also reassures the surgeons, enabling them to operate on high-risk patients.

2   WHICH TYPES OF SURGERY ARE MONITORED AND WHY?

All types of kyphosis, scoliosis, or combinations of these are monitored. Deformity trauma (largely proximal), eg, cervical and myelopathic patients, are also monitored.

The decision as to whether an operation should be monitored is based on several factors.

3   PATIENTS NOT REQUIRING ANY FORM OF MONITORING

The following are instances where monitoring may be considered unnecessary. These include cases in which the detection of monitoring changes would not affect the course of surgery or previous quality of life.

- Spinal tumors where surgical tumor removal is necessary regardless of neurological changes.
- Patients with poor neurological function preoperatively, such as severe sensory motor disability with incontinence and the inability to walk.
- Low-risk cases where the spinal cord is not thought to be at risk, eg, laminectomy and anterior discectomy.

4   WHAT IS MONITORED?

4.1   SOMATOSENSORY-EVOKED POTENTIALS (SSEPs)

The recording of cortical or cervical responses following electrical stimulation of a peripheral sensory nerve is routinely practiced. This allows the sensory pathways in the spinal cord to be monitored continuously and thus gives an indication of the integrity of the spinal cord. Some centers use a method involving epidural recording of the sensory pathways. However, this method of recording does not allow monitoring of all types of surgery. SSEP monitoring does not have any contraindications.

4.2   MOTOR-EVOKED POTENTIALS (MEPs)

Peripheral responses are recorded from several muscles in the hands, legs, and feet following electrical stimulus of the cerebral cortex. This allows the motor pathways in the spinal cord to be monitored, thus giving an indication of the integrity of the motor tracts of the spinal cord.

We currently do not undertake MEP monitoring in the following patients:

- past medical history of seizures or unexplained blackouts
- previous head injury sustained where the patient lost consciousness
- metallic implants or any other devices within their skull, eg, aneurysm clips
- unstable fractures.

4.3   LEVEL OF MUSCLE RELAXANT

The level of muscle relaxant is also monitored to aid in the interpretation of both SSEPs and MEPs. The measurements obtained then provide an indication of the patient's degree of muscle relaxation. If muscle relaxation is too great then it is not possible to record any MEPs. Conversely, if the level of muscle relaxant is too low, the patient's body may jerk each time a stimulus is presented, thereby interfering with the surgical procedure and possibly injuring the patient.

4.4   ELECTRICAL POTENTIALS RECORDED BY THE ELECTROENCEPHALOGRAPH

One or two channels of electroencephalography (EEG) are continuously monitored using a compressed display, eg, cerebral function analyzing monitor (CFAM) [1], or similar. This provides an indication of the effects that anesthetic agents have on the raw EEG, aiding in the interpretation of cortical-evoked potentials.

---

5   HOW ARE THE POTENTIALS MONITORED?

5.1   SSEPs

Electrodes are placed on the skin over a nerve which runs relatively close to the surface (**Fig 1.3-1**).

An electrical pulse is applied across the electrodes and a nerve action potential is generated which then travels along the nerve to the spinal cord, and eventually to the cortex of the brain.

The resulting potentials which are recorded from over the cervical spine area and cortex of the brain are SSEPs. Several SSEPs from two or more electrodes are recorded simultaneously.

Two stimulation sites are routinely used (these must be below the level of surgery):

- posterior tibial nerve at the ankle,
- median nerve at the wrist (used in cervical surgery where the level of surgery is above C7).

The recording sites should then be above the level of surgery:

- cervical—C2, C5, and C7,
- cortex of the brain—differing areas dependant upon which limb is stimulated,
- spinal cord—using epidural electrodes placed on the surface of the spinal cord.

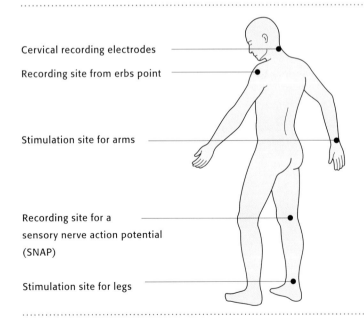

Cervical recording electrodes

Recording site from erbs point

Stimulation site for arms

Recording site for a
sensory nerve action potential
(SNAP)

Stimulation site for legs

Fig 1.3-1
Placement positions for the electrodes.

In addition, a sensory nerve action potential is recorded from behind the knee or over the brachial plexus at erbs point (shoulder)—this checks the function of the stimulator from each limb, ie, if the stimulator stops working then the nerve action potential will be absent (**Fig 1.3-2**).

The clinical physiologist should liaise with the anesthetist throughout the procedure as the recordings obtained are dependent upon numerous factors:

- blood volume,
- blood pressure,
- muscle relaxant,
- anesthetic agents used.

5.1.1 COMMON PROBLEMS ENCOUNTERED

- Diathermy use prevents the accumulation of evoked potentials due to electrical interference.
- Electrical interference from other mains supplied equipment in use within the operating room environment, eg, infusion pumps.
- Electrodes (both stimulating and recording) accidentally becoming disconnected during the procedure.

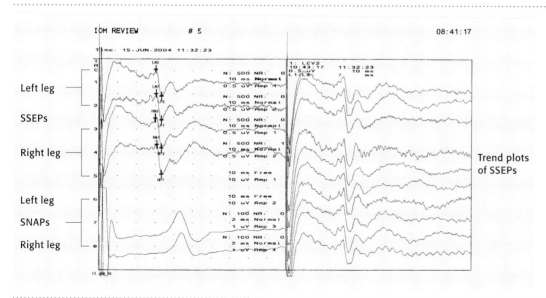

Fig 1.3-2
Trace example of SSEPs.

5.1.2 SSEP CHANGES DURING SPINAL CORD MONITORING

The criteria which is most often adopted to define a significant change in the SSEP during monitoring is the percentage decrease in the amplitude of the response.

The amplitude of SSEPs vary naturally from one recording to the next, therefore many departments have adopted a criterion of 50% amplitude reduction as a significant change, before notifying the surgeon (**Fig 1.3-3**).

This criteria occasionally produces false positive results where no clinical deficit is apparent postoperatively.

5.1.3 DISADVANTAGES

As the surface SSEP is a very small electrical potential (typically 0.1–1.0 µV), approximately 500 runs are averaged together to obtain a visible response. This process takes over 1 minute to achieve each response, which can be frustrating when determining whether the response is absent.

Cortical potentials are more sensitive to changes in blood pressure and the anesthetic agents being used, therefore at times they have a more marked variability in amplitude than potentials recorded from the spinal cord.

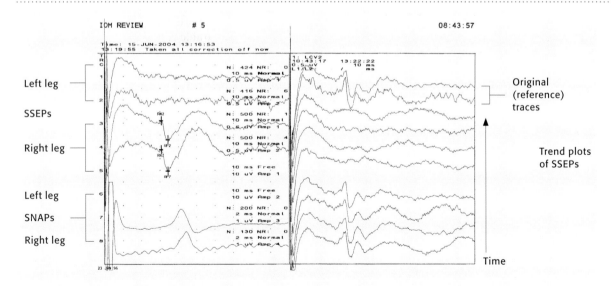

Fig 1.3-3
Trace examples—SSEPs absent trend.

Due to the low amplitude of surface SSEPs the patient should be given an adequate amount of muscle relaxant from the anesthetist throughout the procedure, otherwise random electrical potentials generated from the muscle fibers may mask the SSEP.

When epidural recording electrodes are used, they must be inserted by the surgeon during surgery when the spine is exposed. Responses are usually larger when recording epidurally as opposed to recording from surface electrodes, and therefore acquisition of these responses should be shorter.

Epidural recording electrodes are more likely to be accidentally dislodged during surgery, thus making recordings impossible until the electrode is repositioned.

A direct comparison of recordings is not possible once the electrode has been repositioned, as the epidural electrode will not be in exactly the same position as before. Epidural recording electrodes are not possible during surgery involving the high cervical region.

SSEPs monitor the afferent volley in the posterior columns. Selective damage to the motor pathways cannot be detected using SSEPs alone. The ability to monitor the descending motor tracts is a desirable addition to monitoring SSEPs.

5.2   MEPS

Two silver disk electrodes, which are coated with a layer of silver chloride, are applied over the motor cortex on the right and left hemispheres. These electrodes then act as stimulators.

The recording electrodes are placed over the surface of a muscle (using surface electrodes) or subdermally (using subdermal needle electrodes). Muscle groups typically recorded include:

• abductor allicus (AH)	feet
• tibialis anterior (TA)	legs
• quadriceps (Q)	legs
• abductor digitorum hallicus (ADH)	hands
• abductor digitorum minimi (ADM)	hands

A pulsed stimulus of around 4 pulses at a range of 300–700 V with an interstimulus interval of 2 ms is routinely used, dependant upon a response being recorded from the electrodes. As the response is being recorded from muscles (and not nerves as in SSEPs), the amplitude of the response is much larger, ie, several millivolts, and therefore only one pulsed stimulus is required to obtain a measurable response.

The responses recorded (**Fig 1.3-4**) vary in both shape and size, and only the amplitude is measured. Latency is not measured. Only when the responses become absent and no longer reproducible is the surgeon informed.

5.2.1 DISADVANTAGES

The MEPs are very sensitive to anesthetics used as well as any changes made during the procedure. Total intravenous anesthesia using propofol in combination with an opioid, eg, fentanyl, is now an established technique and in conjunction with controlled hypotension provides good monitoring conditions to record compound muscle action potentials throughout surgery. At the time of writing, there are concerns regarding the use of propofol during anesthesia of young children, and therefore MEPs are not recorded during these cases.

5.2.2 MEP CHANGES DURING SURGERY

As there is a much greater variation in waveforms recorded from the motor system, the criteria used is simply whether the MEP waveform is present or not.

5.3   LEVEL OF MUSCLE RELAXANT (TRAIN-OF-FOUR)

This is measured by stimulating a nerve, eg, posterior tibial at the ankle, on four occasions (each stimulus is only a few seconds apart) and recording the amplitude of the muscle potentials generated from each of these stimuli, eg, abductor hallicus, at the foot (**Fig 1.3-5**). The amplitude of the resulting traces is then measured and plotted as a trend graph showing the amplitude (bar graph) and latency (line above) of each response recorded.

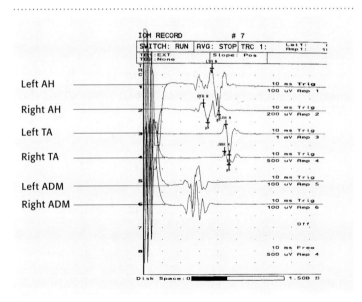

Fig 1.3-4
Trace example of MEPs.

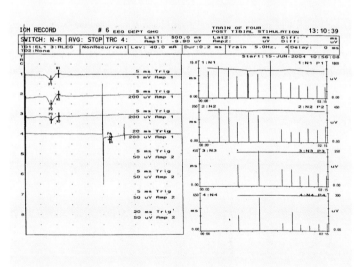

Fig 1.3-5
Trace example train-of-four.

6   BIBLIOGRAPHY

1.   **Maynard DE** (1979) Development of the CFM: the Cerebral Function Analysing Monitor (CFAM). *Ann Anesthesiol Fr;* 20(3):253–255.

5.4   CEREBRAL FUNCTION ANALYZING MONITOR

Cerebral function analyzing monitor (CFAM) records one or two channels of EEG (**Fig 1.3-6**) which is continuously monitored throughout surgery, providing an indication of the effects that anesthetic agents have on the raw EEG. This is an aid to the interpretation of cortical-evoked potentials.

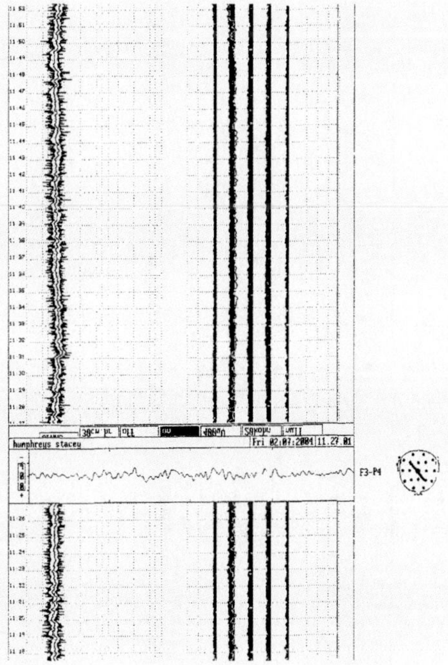

Fig 1.3-6
Trace example of CFAM.

1   GENERAL KNOWLEDGE FOR SPINE SURGERY
1.4   GRAFTS IN SPINE SURGERY

1.4   GRAFTS IN SPINE SURGERY

1   INTRODUCTION

A bone graft is a section of autograft, allograft, or graft substitutes required to improve function or strengthen an area of the skeletal system. It can be placed in many locations in the spine, eg, to promote fusion, to correct deformity when regaining height to spinal column, replace fractured or diseased bone, and to help to support instrumentation. Surgery where bones grow together biologically and develop into a solid mass is considered a success. They can be defined in several ways, as shown below [1]:

- donor site,
- grafts,
- graft substitutes,
- graft enhancers,
- osteoconductive,
- osteoinductive,
- osteogenic.

2   DONOR SITE

The donor site is the area from which the bone graft is taken (harvested), eg, iliac crest. In many cases this is the preferred method and seen as the gold standard for lumbar fusion. This graft contains two properties which aid fusion osteogenicity and osteoconduction. It is estimated that generally 15% of the bone cells survive transplantation.

3   DEFINITIONS

Graft

A graft is a tissue or substance that is placed at a site different from its site of origin. In the spine, a graft is generally the patient's own bone. Bone from another person or substances are used to extend or enhance bony fusion. Other surgical grafts include skin, liver, cornea, kidneys, etc.

Graft substitute

A graft substitute is a material capable of achieving fusion rates equal to or greater than autogenous bone without the need for autograft [2].

Graft extender

This is a substance that, when added to autograft, allows for the fusion of more levels or the use of less autograft, and results in a rate of fusion equal to that of autogenous bone.

Graft enhancer

A graft enhancer, when added to autogenous bone, yields a higher rate of fusion than autogenous bone alone.

Osteoconductive

Osteoconductive is the ability of a material to act as a scaffold for the attachment of osteogenic cells.

Osteoinductive

Biological stimuli from growth factors and cytokines—such as bone morphogenetic protein (BMP), transforming growth factor beta (TGF-β), insulin-like growth factor (IGF), and platelet-derived growth factor (PDGF)—are used to stimulate osteoblastic progenitor cells to proliferate and differentiate into bone.

Osteogenic

Osteogenic cells must be present either within the graft (autograft), transplanted into the graft at surgery (bone marrow aspirate), or able to migrate into the graft from surrounding tissue (adjacent bone, periosteum, muscle, fat, or connective tissue).

4   GRAFTS, GRAFT SUBSTITUTES, AND GRAFT ENHANCERS

There are many grafts and graft counterparts available, both biological and nonbiological. The decision of which to use is determined by the surgeon's preference, as each patient's skeletal bone quality varies.

4.1   BIOLOGICAL

- Cortical
  This is often allograft (such as fibula) that is used for its mechanical strength in cervical and lumbar spine when trauma, tumor, and degenerative conditions require anterior column support.

- Cancellous
  This is the less strong, central part of a living bone that is used as a graft when structural support is not as important as osteoinductive and osteoconductive potential, such as in posterolateral fusion in posterior deformity (scoliosis) cases. The greater trochanter is normally an excellent source for harvesting cancellous bone; it can be taken from the patient's own iliac crest anteriorly or posteriorly from the wings of the ilium thus allowing the crest to remain intact.

- Autogenous
  This is graft originating from the skeleton of the same individual into whom it is to be placed. When the graft is required for lumbar anterior surgery, a core of bone can be taken from the vertebral body at the level above the defect. This core can then be replaced with a bone substitute.

- Allograft
  By definition, this originates from another being of the same species and is commonly cadaveric. It is prepared by the processes of freeze drying or fresh frozen. Freeze drying allows a long storage life and decreased antigenicity at the expense of mechanical strength. Fresh frozen graft maintains its strength. Cadaveric allograft is sterilized (low dose irradiation, ethanol, etc) which renders it primarily osteoconductive, as most of its osteoinductive capabilities are lost with the sterilization and preparation procedures.

- Xenograft
  This is graft taken from a different species.

5   APPLICATIONS OF GRAFTS IN SPINE SURGERY

4.2   NONBIOLOGICAL

- Ceramics
  Ceramics are formed by heating and pressurizing calcium phosphates. Tricalcium phosphate and hydroxyapatite are the most commonly used ceramics in spinal fusion. They are safe and biocompatible. However, they are brittle and have low fracture resistance, and therefore are not generally used in load-bearing situations. The porous structure of the ceramics allows vascularization and a large surface area to which osteogenic cells can adhere.

- Dematerialized bone matrix (DBM)
  DBM is what is left when the bone mineral is extracted from bone by acids. It is made up of collagen, various (noncollagenous) proteins, and growth factors. Amongst these growth factors is BMP. Numerous types of DBM are available including gel, putty, and sheet fibers. It is generally used as a graft extender.

- Bone morphogenetic protein (BMP)
  BMPs are a family of at least 24 related growth factors within the TGF superfamily. They are able to stimulate bone formation by causing pluripotent precursor cells to differentiate into bone-forming cells (osteoblasts and chondroblasts).

5.1   CERVICAL

- Posterior/posterolateral: normally autogenous cancellous bone with occasional extenders.
- Anterior: often tricortical corticocancellous autograft from the iliac crest. Also metal/mesh cages can be used with or without plates.

5.2   THORACIC

- Posterior/posterolateral: most commonly used in deformity surgery in children. Again autogenous cancellous graft is used but extenders are not always required in children due to their ability to fuse readily.
- Anterior: mesh cages filled with autogenous graft with extender can be used.

5.3   LUMBAR

- Posterior/posterolateral: normally autogenous cancellous bone with occasional extenders/enhancers.
- Posterior lumbar interbody fusion (PLIF) utilizes the posterolateral graft and an interbody graft (eg, cortico-cancellous, autogenous, allograft, enhancers, extenders) or interbody cages. Both grafts are put in from the posterior approach.
- Anterior lumbar interbody fusion (ALIF): as above but the interbody graft is placed from the front with an anterior approach.
- Transforaminal lumbar interbody fusion (TLIF): as for PLIF but a different operative technique, with a transforaminal approach to the disc.

6   PROBLEMS WITH GRAFTS

Donor site complications

The incidence of donor site complications in spine surgery is significant. Complication rates have been noted to range from 6–25%. Noted complications are painful scarring, increased blood loss, donor site pain, prolonged rehabilitation time, pelvic fracture, neuropathy, and infection [3].

Volume

In spine surgery there is often a disparity between the amount of graft required and the amount that can be harvested from the local bone/iliac crests (pelvis). This is why graft extenders are used.

Physical problems

Autogenous graft, allograft, and ceramics can collapse, reabsorb or change position after implantation. Outside of the spine this may be little more than an annoyance but within the spine this may result in nerve root or cord compression with serious consequences. It is for these reasons that metal cages have been designed to act as spacers/containers and allow fusion to progress around or through them while at the same time avoiding graft spillage into the spinal canal.

Nonunion

Fusion is not guaranteed with autogenous graft. The more spinal levels involved in the fusion, the lesser the chance of successful fusion. It is for this reason that other technologies have been utilized to extend and enhance the chance of fusion.

7   BIBLIOGRAPHY

1. **Yu WD, Roenbeck KM** (2003) Bone graft substitutes and expanders for the spine. *Contemporary Spine Surgery;* 4 (11): 81–87.
2. **Khan SN, Sama A, Sandhu HS** (2001) Bone graft substitutes in spine surgery. *Curr Opin Orthop ;*12:216–222.
3. **Cotler JM, Star AM** (1990) Complications in spinal fusion. *Cotler JM, Cotler HB (eds), Spine Fusions: Science and Technique.* New York: Springer-Verlag, 90–99.

PATHOLOGY OF THE SPINE

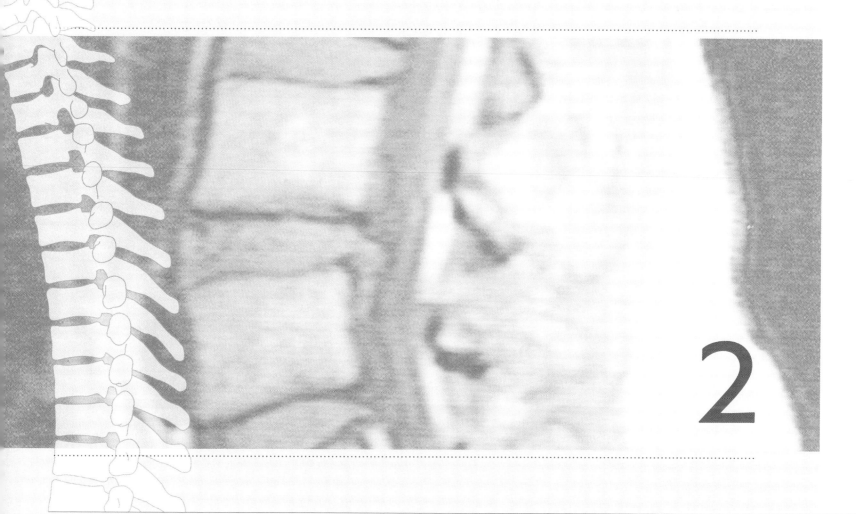

2

2 PATHOLOGY OF THE SPINE

2.1   THE PAINFUL SPINE

1   INTRODUCTION

The spine has three functions:

- It transmits load.
- It allows movement.
- It protects the spinal cord and acts as a conduit for nerves to the body, the arms, and the legs.

The spine consists of a column of individual vertebrae with soft discs between. The vertebrae individually are blocks of bone, with a hole in the middle, to which are attached ligaments and muscles. The discs are precisely that, a disc-shaped soft structure, soft in the centre, and with a thick fibrous outer portion. When these structures are joined together there is therefore a canal, in which the spinal cord lies, from the 1st cervical vertebra to about the 1st lumbar vertebra, and then below this the canal contains the nerves of the cauda equina, which go to the legs, bladder, and bowels.

Malfunction of the spine due to injury, degeneration, infection, or deformity may cause pain from the spine itself, or from the nerve structures within it.

Operations are carried out on the spine for a number of quite different reasons:

- to correct deformity, either congenital, due to growth (scoliosis and kyphosis) or due to trauma,
- to relieve pain caused by malfunction of the spine,
- to relieve pain caused by irritation or compression of the nerves and spinal cord within the spine.

This chapter will not discuss the role of surgery in correcting spinal deformity, except insofar as deformity may be associated with pain. Spinal deformity, especially scoliosis in children and young adults, is usually painless, but in the older adult deformity may be painful. There is one type of deformity in adolescents and adults which may be painful, spondylolisthesis (see 3.4 Spondylolisthesis, in this chapter).

In considering the role of surgery in treating back pain it is vital at the outset to distinguish between:

- pain in the back due to malfunction of the spine itself, so-called mechanical back pain (or activity-related back pain),
- pain due to disturbance of the nerves within the spine, so-called neurological pain, commonly producing not only back pain but pain in the buttocks and legs.

One confusing factor is that mechanical back pain alone, with no evidence of nerve irritation, can produce leg pain. This is known as referred pain, and commonly does not extend below the knees. The importance of recognizing this type of pain is that surgery which solves the mechanical malfunction of the spine will cure the pain, and the spinal canal nerves need not be disturbed.

Clearly, if we are planning to operate on the spine for back pain due to spinal malfunction, it is essential that we know the cause of the pain. In other words, how does spinal malfunction produce pain? It is easy to understand why fractures, acute trauma, and infections within the spine cause pain, as they lead to an acute inflammatory reaction, and we know that is painful. However, most mechanical back pain is not associated with an inflammatory reaction and the cause of the pain is ill understood.

2   REASONS FOR MECHANICAL BACK PAIN

2.1   THE SPINAL DISC AND DEGENERATION

The spinal segment consists of two vertebrae and the disc between them. The disc is the structure that allows movement and transmits load. It is postulated that mechanical back pain is due to disturbance in the function of this segment.

Although mechanical back pain can occur even when the intervertebral disc is apparently normal, back pain is usually associated with degenerate or injured discs. Disc degeneration is the anatomical disruption of the normal disc structure. It is thought to be largely genetic, but influenced by injury. The inside of the disc (the nucleus) becomes fibrous and fragmented and the outer ring of the disc (the annulus) develops tears. The disc ceases to function normally. It allows an abnormal pattern of movement and transmits load irregularly over the vertebrae. It also develops abnormal chemicals and nerves within it (normally it has no nerves). The mixture of mechanical and chemical causes from the abnormal disc are thought to be key factors in the causation of pain.

Pain may come from ligaments which are abnormally stressed, and muscles which have to react differently due to the abnormal mechanical behavior of the disc. The general term instability is often used, meaning a dysfunction of the segment (vertebra-disc-vertebra) but it must be appreciated that this does not mean that the segment is unstable like an unstable knee or shoulder. Most commonly the segment is stiffer than normal.

The cause of mechanical low back pain remains largely mis-understood, which is one reason why surgery to treat it is often empirical rather than based on sound pathological knowledge. Many very degenerate discs produce no pain, and mechanical studies of the spine have not correlated any pattern of abnormal movement with pain.

2.2   BACK PAIN

Nearly half of the adult population suffers from back pain of sufficient severity for them to consult their doctor at some time. The severity and persistence of the pain determines whether surgery is a reasonable option. Spine surgery is a very invasive procedure, has both morbidity and mortality risks, and is uncertain in outcome. Hence, back pain must be disabling and severe for surgery to be even considered. Careful judgment is required to determine whether surgery is appropriate for any one individual. We cannot measure pain directly and have to rely on the disability it produces; this is dependant on the psychology of the individual. Accordingly, a crucial element in deciding whether surgery is appropriate is a comprehensive evaluation of all the psychological, social, and economic factors which cause an individual's pain, which produce that degree of disability. Obviously, surgical treatment will not resolve these factors.

Although back pain is often associated with a degenerate disc, a patient may have a degenerate disc but have no pain. In this instance, plain x-rays are often not very helpful in determining exactly where pain is coming from. Magnetic resonance imaging (MRI) does show the degree of disc degeneration very accurately, and will identify nerve compression very precisely, but again a degenerate disc may not necessarily be the cause of back pain. Diagnosing the source of pain and appreciating its significance in a patient is a very uncertain process, which is one reason why surgery for mechanical back pain is somewhat unsatisfactory—we do not always know the cause, the site, and the true severity. Thus, it is critical that prior to advising surgery, we know all we can about the pain and the patient, and back this up with thorough investigations to accurately determine the site and cause of the pain.

While we have little understanding of the cause of mechanical back pain, we have a greater knowledge of pain which is due to neurological compression. Neurological compression primarily causes leg and buttock pain, but combined with this can be back pain. The development of MRI now allows very precise pictures to be created of the neural elements within the spine, and we can make a fairly precise diagnosis of where nerves within the spinal canal are compressed and to what degree of compression. Although plain x-rays may allow us to deduce where nerves are likely to be compressed, the MRI gives much more precise information—thus, the MRI is the investigation method of choice.

3   NEUROLOGICAL COMPRESSIVE DISORDERS REQUIRING SURGERY

3.1   DISC HERNIATION (SLIPPED DISC)

Disc herniation is a disorder where a portion of the disc or shock absorber between the vertebrae protrudes and presses on a nerve. When it occurs in the lower back, nerves leading to the leg are pressed. By simply asking the patient where the pain is felt we can determine to a considerable extent which disc is protruding. Pain down the back of the leg suggests it is the disc between the L5 and the S1 vertebrae (sacrum), if the back and side of the leg are painful, it is the disc above (L4/5), and if it is the front of the leg it is the disc above that (L3/4). Often, a patient will give a history that their back suddenly "went", and within a few hours or over the next day or so they suddenly felt severe leg pain. This is commonly called sciatica, as most usually it is one of the two lower discs that protrude cause pain down the back of the leg. In most cases the disc shrinks, and the patient improves. However, if it does not improve over the next few weeks or is very severe, then the protruding bit of disc may be removed surgically. The operation is often called a laminectomy, because previously the lamina that is the back of the vertebrae was removed to gain access. Nowadays, this operation may also be called a discectomy, although only a small portion of the disc is removed. The procedure simply goes between the lamina and takes just the ligament flavum away. Only the protruding section of disc is removed, and any loose disc within the disc space. The whole disc weighs about 20 g, and usually the most determined surgeon will only remove about 2 to 3 g. This is an operation for leg pain due to nerve entrapment, and is not an operation for back pain. Patients need only to stay in hospital for a day or so, and should aim to get back to normal activity in a few weeks. The back is not destabilized. Early active physiotherapy is good, as it gives the patient confidence to get back to full activity as quickly as possible.

3.2   CAUDA EQUINA LESION

On occasion, the disc protrusion is so great that it squeezes all the nerves in the cauda equina (the bag containing all the nerves to the legs, bowels, and bladder). Whereas a disc protrusion pressing on one nerve is not a surgical emergency, if it presses on all the nerves, then it is. The patient presents with acute back pain and complains of difficulty with passing urine. If questioned and examined they will have numbness around their buttocks, and the anal sphincter will be lax. They may or may not have sciatica. In these cases, the operation has to be undertaken as soon as possible, most certainly within 48 hours from the start of the compression, lest bowel and bladder function not recover, and the patient be left incontinent of urine and feces. Further, the patient may suffer impotency if a man, or complete vaginal and clitoral loss of sensation if a woman.

Thus, if a patient arrives with urine retention and/or a numb buttock, then it is a surgical emergency. The patient will require an immediate MRI scan to diagnose where the disc protrusion is, and to exclude a non compressive neurological disorder such as a transverse myelitis of the spinal cord.

3.3   SPINAL STENOSIS

In older people, disc degeneration and the narrowing of disc space can lead to a reduction of space for the nerves in the lower back. This interferes with nerve function and also blood supply to the nerve. The patient complains that as they walk they get sciatica and often back pain. It is relieved if they bend forward, as this increases the space within the spinal canal. This syndrome is often called spinal elucidation. Elucidation means to limp when one walks, as the Emperor Claudius did, hence the use of the term claudication. It can be due to a shortage of blood to the legs, arterial elucidation, or spinal stenosis. It is said that the vascular claudicant stops to relieve the pain, and stands upright and lights a cigarette (they are usually cigarette smokers), while the spinal claudicant stops and pretends to pick up a cigarette butt, bending to relieve their pain.

In this disorder, surgery is not urgent and careful investigation with both MRI and CT scanning are required to identify precisely where the stenosis occurs. If they are significantly disabled, especially with regard to their walking distance, then more space can be made in the spine by taking the lamina and the ligament between the lamina away (the ligamentum flavum). This is major surgery compared to an operation for a disc herniation, as the patient will usually be much older, and often has other comorbidities. They recover slowly, as the injury to the spine is greater. If any hematomas develop around the surgical site during the postoperative stage, they may develop a cauda equina lesion, and urgent reoperation may be required. Postoperatively, the function of the bowel and bladder, as well as the sensation around the buttocks, must be frequently and very carefully assessed.

3.4   SPONDYLOLISTHESIS

This cumbersome term covers a variety of deformities with very different causes, in which one vertebra slips forward in relation to the one below. The reason for the slipping forward is the important fact, and treatment is related to that rather than the slipping forward. In middle-aged people (more commonly women), this can occur due to osteoarthritis of the facet joints of the spine, and associated degenerative disc disease. This is called degenerative spondylolisthesis. It can lead to back pain, or the syndrome of spinal stenosis. It is an important cause of spinal stenosis, but spinal stenosis can occur with degenerative disease alone, and with no slipping of the vertebrae. If, however, the cause of the stenosis is degenerative spondylolisthesis, then it is necessary to decompress the nerves in the spine, as well as do a fusion operation. Therefore, this group of patients requires major surgery. The slip is not progressive—so such surgery is by no means essential, and patients with spinal stenosis and degenerative spondylolisthesis may be observed for years with no further progression of their symptoms. The reason for operating is severity of symptoms, not fear for the future.

4   INDICATIONS FOR SURGERY

4.1   DISC DEGENERATION

As indicated in the precious paragraphs we are very uncertain of causes of so called mechanical back pain. It is accepted that in many cases it is related to degenerative disc disease. However, perhaps only 5% of back pain requires surgical treatment.

The indications for treatment are the severity and chronicity of the pain. No one with mechanical back pain for less than 2 years should be operated upon, as most back pain does improve over a two year period. If we were more confident of the cause, and of the success rates of back pain operations, one could advocate earlier intervention. In a sense every operation for mechanical back pain is an experiment.

The spine is a series of joints. We know that in the past painful joints could be cured if we stiffened them; arthrodesis of the knee, hip, and ankle, and indeed any painful joint. This was a common procedure in the last century until joint replacement became possible. It was argued that the painful spine could also be cured by stiffening. However, two major problems with this procedure were: which of the many joints was the source of the pain, and could we with any certainty fuse the joint or joints?

With these two points in mind, a very definite series of assessments must be made when deciding if a patient with backache should have an operation:

- Is the patient's condition serious enough to warrant major surgery which may make him/her worse, and in which the success rate is only in the region of 50–60%?
- Do we know which segments of the spine are the cause of the pain?
- How can we ensure that we fuse the spine with certainty?

With regard to the first assessment, careful clinical assessment is vital, as is a full appraisal of the social and economic environment of the patient. For example, a man might have moderate back pain, but is managing to cope with his job. If a spinal fusion is performed, he may be off work for some months. Furthermore, his employers may not re-employ him knowing that he has had a back operation. Sadly, it is universally acknowledged that a person who is involved in litigation concerning an injury that produced their back pain is much less likely to do well with surgical treatment.

Plain x-rays are not of great value in considering the second assessment, as marked degenerative change can be present and not cause pain. We have to both identify structural change (using MRI and CT and plain films) and demonstrate that the morphological change is painful. Clinical examination can give some guidance in this assessment, and we may use discography. This is a procedure where a needle is introduced into the suspected painful disc, and fluid is injected. If this reproduces the pain, then that is the segment that is causative. However, despite the apparently simple logic of this, it is in fact a somewhat imprecise exercise.

For the third assessment, the means of achieving a solid fusion has altered each decade since the 1950s.

Initially, bone (taken from the iliac crest) was placed around the segments to be fused, and the patient placed in a plaster bed. The plaster bed was eventually replaced by a plaster cast, which was also despensed with, and no external support was used at all. At this time, rigid metal rods and plates were used to internally hold the segments together. However, clinical results did not improve despite the improvements in fixation methods. Hence it was felt that the operation needed a more serious approach. Using this method, the abdomen was opened, and the disc taken out. The disc was replaced initially by bone, and later by metal cages. At the same time, the spine was fixed from behind with metal rods. Nevertheless, it became clear that despite achieving almost 100% fusion, the clinical results remained very similar to those achieved using bone alone, with no fixation, and only anterior instrumentation.

Fusion improves the condition of a significant number of people with disabling low back pain. Nonetheless, it is unpredictable, and every surgeon feels his technique gives the best chance to his patients. All surgeons agree that patient selection is critical, and that postoperative rehabilitation is vital. Despite being very major surgery, it is vital that patients are mobilized as quickly as possible after surgery and proceed with early energetic rehabilitation.

4.2   SPONDYLOLISTHESIS

There are various types of spondylolisthesis. Degenerative spondylolisthesis, seen in older people and the other important type of spondylolisthesis the so-called lytic spondylolisthesis, which occurs due to a defect in the back of the vertebrae, allowing the vertebrae to slip forward in some patients. It is also called a lysis or pars defect. It is acquired probably at about 12 years of age, during the rapid growth period, and the intense physical activities of a child at that age. It commonly causes no pain. It is present in some 5% of the population, and may remain symptomless throughout life. However, sometimes in adolescents it can become painful and be associated with a major slip. Fusion in young patients is usually very successful. Although it may be symptomless in adolescence and early adulthood, it can become symptomatic in later life, especially after an injury. Fusion in these older patients is no more likely to be successful than fusion for degenerative disc disease.

On occasion, this type of spondylolisthesis can produce focal nerve root compression in later life—a spinal stenosis affecting just one nerve root. Surgery, involving decompression alone, for this disorder is very successful.

4.3   SCOLIOSIS

Scoliosis is not a cause of back pain in adolescents and young adults. However in older people, scoliosis can occur as a result of degenerative disc disease, and such patients may require surgical treatment. These are patients where fusion is necessary to correct the deformity, and where the use of internal fixation is necessary.

5   OTHER CAUSES OF BACK PAIN

It must be appreciated that there are other spinal disorders that produce back pain, such as tumors, infection, and trauma.

5.1   TUMORS IN THE BONE OF THE SPINE

Most spinal tumors are secondary tumors, and the basis of treatment is to control the primary tumor with systemic treatment, and stabilize the spine. It was often thought that spinal secondaries were intrinsically painful. It is now recognized that most of the pain, unless there is nerve or cord compression is due to the spine essentially being fractured. Hence we now very actively stabilize the spine with internal fixation if someone has a painful metastasis producing bony collapse. This is very important in breast carcinoma, where many women may live for years after their spine has been stabilized, and the primary tumor brought under control with drugs and hormones.

5.2   INFECTION

The spine can contract bacterial infections, either in the bone (osteomyelitis) or in the disc (discitis). The latter is very uncommon, as there is no blood supply to the normal disc to allow bacteria entry. Discitis may however follow surgery to the disc or discography. The patient is in very severe pain; just jogging the bed produces screams. This diagnosis must be considered if a patient seems to be in excessive pain after disc surgery. Most spinal infection can be dealt with using antibiotics alone, but in the rare instance that pus has formed, it must be "let out". After appropriate imaging, the site of the pus can be identified, and the spine opened to evacuate the abscess.

Spinal tuberculosis

This is a very critical spinal infection, as it leads to deformity and can cause paralysis. Because it is so subacute, it will mimic ordinary mechanical back pain, and often it may be treated as such initially. With the advent of MRI, diagnosis can now be made before any bony changes are seen. Although most tuberculosis is sensitive to available chemotherapeutic agents, surgery is often part of the management. Deformity can be dealt with, and any tuberculous material can be removed. Such surgery is almost invariably performed through the abdomen or chest, as it is the disc and vertebrae that are infected, and access to these is clearly much easier from the front.

6 SUGGESTIONS FOR FURTHER READING

Bartley R, Coffey P (2001) *Management of low back pain in primary care.* Oxford: Butterworth Heinemann.
McCulloch J (1986) *McNab's Backache.* 2nd ed. Baltimore: Williams and Wilkins.
Tsuji H (1990) *Comprehensive atlas of lumbar spine surgery.* St Louis: Mosby Year Book.
Yonenobu K, Ono K, Takemitsu Y (1993) *Lumbar fusion and stabilization.* Berlin Heidelberg: Springer-Verlag.

2.2 DEGENERATIVE DISC DISEASE

1 INTRODUCTION

Back pain is a major public health problem in industrialized western society. It results in suffering, and distress to patients and their close families. It affects a large number of people, the prevalence rate ranging from 12% to 35% with about 10% becoming chronically disabled [1]. This causes a large burden on the economic community with medical costs, insurance, and lost production (eg, an estimated at £12 billion per year in the UK) [1].

Back pain is associated with intervertebral disc degeneration. Disc degeneration can be asymptomatic in many cases, but can also be associated with disc herniation leading to brachalgia, sciatica, or cauda equina syndrome. Degeneration alters disc height and therefore the biomechanics of the spinal column, as well as affecting the surrounding muscle and ligament behavior. Sequela of long-term disc degeneration is spinal stenosis, more commonly seen in the elderly; its incidence is rising sharply with the current demographic changes and an increasing aged population.

Discs degenerate before other surrounding musculoskeletal tissues; the first unequivocal sign of degeneration is seen in the age group 11–16 years [2]. Studies have shown that about 20% of people in their teens have discs with mild signs of degeneration; degeneration increases rapidly with age, especially in males, so that about 10% of 50-year-old discs and about 60% of 70-year-old discs are severely degenerate [3].

2   MORPHOLOGY OF THE INTERVERTEBRAL DISC

2.1   NORMAL DISC

The intervertebral disc lies between the two vertebral bodies and links them together. They are not true joints as such but represent 1/3 of spinal column height. They play a role in its mechanical function as they transmit loads arising from body weight and muscle activity. They allow flexibility in three planes:

- flexion,
- lateral bending,
- torsion.

They are about 7–10 mm in height and 4 cm in the anteroposterior diameter. The disc itself is a complex structure with a thick outer ring of fibrous cartilage named the annulus fibrosus, which surrounds an inner gelatinous core named the nucleus pulposus. The cartilaginous vertebral end plates sandwich the nucleus pulposus. The cartilaginous end plate is a thin horizontal layer usually less than 1 mm in thickness and formed from hyaline cartilage.

The disc-vertebral body interface is formed by this end plate. The collagen fibers within it run horizontal and parallel to the vertebra, with the fibers entering the disc.

The normal healthy adult disc has few if any blood vessels, but it does have some nerve fibers. These are normally seen in the outer lamellae of the annulus which terminate in proprioceptors. The end plate is normally avascular and aneural in the healthy adult disc.

2.2   DEGENERATED DISC

With growth and skeletal maturation the boundary between the outer annulus and inner nucleus becomes more indistinct, and with increasing age the nucleus generally becomes more fibrotic and less gel-like. This ageing process causes changes in the morphology, with the disc becoming more disorganized. There is resultant cleft formation with fissures forming within the disc, particularly seen in the nucleus. Nerves and blood vessels are seen with increased frequency with degeneration of the disc. The morphological changes associated with disc degeneration were reviewed by Boos et al [2], who demonstrated an age-associated change in morphology, with discs from individuals as young as 2 years having some mild cleft formation in the nucleus. With increased age there is an increased incidence of degenerative change with cell death, mucous degeneration, cell proliferation and annular tears. The difficulty arises in the differentiation of pathological changes from ageing.

3   THE EFFECT OF DISC DEGENERATION ON DISC FUNCTION AND PATHOLOGY

The loss of proteoglycan in disc degeneration has a major effect on the disc's ability in load bearing. As proteoglycan is lost, the osmotic pressure in the disc falls and the disc is less able to maintain hydration under loading. Degenerate discs therefore have a lower water content than normal age-matched discs, and when loaded lose height as a result of fluid loss, allowing the discs to bulge. The matrix disorganization and loss of proteoglycan have other important effects on the biomechanics; because of the loss of hydration, the degenerate discs no longer behave hydrostatically under loading.

Stress concentrations along the end plate or in the annulus may result from loading of the degenerate disc and this has been associated with discogenic pain produced by provocative discography [4].

Such major changes in disc behavior strongly influence other spinal structures and may affect their individual function and predispose them to injury and become a source of pain. With rapid loss of height under loading, the apophyseal joints of the motion segment may be subject to abnormal loads and develop osteoarthritic changes. Loss of disc height can also affect other structures; affecting the tensile forces in the ligamentum flavum and hence causing remodeling and thickening. As the ligament loses its elasticity it may bulge into the spinal canal leading to spinal stenosis, a condition seen increasingly with ageing.

The increased vascular and neural ingrowth seen in the degenerate disc associated with back pain is probably a result of proteoglycan loss as disc aggrecan has been shown to inhibit neural ingrowth [5].

4   DISC HERNIATION

The most common disc disorder seen by spine surgeons is the herniated or prolapsed intervertebral disc. The disc bulges or ruptures posteriorly or more commonly posterolaterally. This will in turn compress the exiting nerve root at that level of the spinal column. Although herniation is thought to be the result of a mechanically-induced rupture, it can only be induced in vitro in normal healthy discs by mechanical forces larger than those that are ever normally encountered; in most experimental tests, the vertebral body will fail first. The disc needs to show some degeneration before the disc can herniate; autopsy studies have shown that sequestration or herniation results from the migration of isolated, degenerate fragments of the nuclear material through preexisting tears in the annulus fibrosus [6].

It has now been shown that herniation-induced pressure on the nerve root cannot singularly be the cause of pain because more than 70% of "normal", asymptomatic people have disc herniations compressing nerve roots without pain.

The current hypothesis is that, in symptomatic people, the nerves are somehow more sensitive to pressure [7]. This may arise as a result of an inflammatory cascade from arachidonic acid through to prostaglandin E2. These molecules and intermediates have been identified from cells of herniated discs [8] and as a result of the close proximity to the nerve root, it may be sensitized. The exact sequence is unknown but patients treated with tumor necrosis factor alpha (TNF-α) antagonists have shown promising results with a decrease in pain [9].

5   ETIOLOGY OF DISC DEGENERATION

Disc degeneration is very difficult to study. Its definition is vague, with diffuse parameters, which prove difficult to quantify. There is no good animal model to investigate it further. One of the most recognized causes of disc degeneration is thought to be failure of the nutrient supply to the disc.

The disc cells require glucose and oxygen for normal function. The disc is large and avascular and the cells rely upon blood vessels at their margins for nutrient supply and waste removal. This pathway is precarious because capillaries originating in the vertebral bodies, penetrating the subchondral plate and ending just above the cartilaginous end plate supply the cells. Nutrients then diffuse through the cartilaginous end plate and extracellular matrix of the nucleus pulposus to the cells, which can be over 8 mm from the capillary vessel. Thus a fall in nutrient supply could ultimately lead to disc degeneration, although there is as yet little evidence.

6   MECHANICAL LOAD, INJURY, AND GENETICS

Abnormal mechanical loads are also thought to provide a cause for disc degeneration. Injury has been suggested as a cause for back problems. This is often work related and is thought to produce structural damage. It is held that such an injury can initiate a chain of events leading to disc degeneration and to clinical symptoms of back pain. Added support for this hypothesis comes from the notion that there is accelerated disc degeneration at adjacent levels to previous fusions. However, this is as yet unproven as a cause, and may just be the result of the natural history.

This injury model has been supported by several epidemiological studies that have found associations between environmental factors and the development of disc degeneration and herniation with heavy physical work, lifting, obesity, and smoking, with the latter being a major risk factor.

Recently, studies have suggested that genetic factors may play an important role in the cause of disc degeneration. Several studies have reported strong familial predisposition for herniation and disc degeneration [10]. Genetic and epidemiological studies suggest that there is a multifactorial nature to disc degeneration.

7   NEW THERAPIES

Current practice is to reduce pain rather than repair the degenerated disc. Treatments are conservative and range from a few days' bed rest, analgesia, and injections to manipulative treatments. Intradiscal treatments have been used but its success is presently being questioned. Disc degeneration-related pain can also be treated surgically by fusion or by discectomy for herniation.

Future therapies will be aimed at aiding repair of the cellular matrix of the disc by inducing disc cells to produce more matrix, or by the use of growth factors to increase the rate of matrix synthesis.

8   BIBLIOGRAPHY

1. **Maniadakis N, Gray A** (2000) The economic burden of back pain in the UK. *Pain;* 84(1):95–103.
2. **Boos N, Weissbach S, Rohrbach H, et al** (2002) Classification of age-related changes in lumbar intervertebral discs: 2002 Volvo Award in basic science. *Spine;* 27(23):2631–2644.
3. **Miller J, Schwatz C, Schultz A** (1998) Lumbar disc degeneration: Correlation with age, sex and spine level in 600 autopsy specimens. *Spine;* 13:173–178.
4. **McNally DS, Shackleford IN, Goodship AE et al** (1996) In vivo stress measurement can predict pain on discography. *Spine;* 21(22):2580–2587.
5. **Johnson WE, Caterson B, Eisenstein SM et al** (2002) Human intervertebral disc aggrecan inhibits nerve growth in vitro. *Arthritis Rheum;* 46(10):2658–2664.
6. **Moore RJ, Vernon-Roberts B, Fraser RD et al** (1996) The origin and fate of herniated lumbar intervertebral disc tissue. *Spine;* 21(18):2149–2155.
7. **Cavanaugh JM** (1995) Neural mechanisms of lumbar pain. *Spine;* 20:1804–1809.
8. **Kang JD, Georgescu HI, McIntyre-Larkin L et al** (1996) Herniated lumbar intervertebral discs spontaneously produced matrix metalloproteinases, nitric oxide, interleukin-6 and prostaglandin E2. *Spine;* 21:271–277.
9. **Korhonen T, Karppinen J, Malmivaara A, et al** (2004) Efficacy of infliximab for disc herniation induced sciatica: one-year follow-up. *Spine;* 29(19):2115–2119.
10. **Heikkila JK, Koskenvuo M, Heliovaara M et al** (1989) Genetic and environmental factors in sciatica. Evidence from a nationwide panel of 9365 adult twin pairs. *Ann Med;* 21(5):393–398.

2.3   THE DEFORMED SPINE

1   INTRODUCTION

A deformed spine can be found in two distinct groups of patients, children and older adults. It is more commonly found in children, where it is often seen for no obvious reason (idiopathic). In older adults it is secondary to degeneration ("wear and tear" or spondylosis). There are two types of deformity: scoliosis and kyphosis. In adults there can also be lateral translation due to degeneration or a forward or backward slip (spondylolisthesis). Spondylolisthesis can also occur in children (secondary to a spondylolysis).

Scoliosis is routinely defined as a lateral curvature of the spine in the coronal plane [1]. Scoliosis is pathological when the lateral curvature exceeds 10° as measured by the Cobb method on standing posteroanterior (not anteroposterior) x-rays. Below 10° it is classed as spinal asymmetry which is not pathological. The prevalence of curves greater than 10° is approximately 25 in 1,000, with a 1.4:1 female-to-male ratio in this group. The prevalence of curves greater than 30° is 1–3 in 1,000 but a 10:1 female-to-male ratio in this group [2].

The definition of scoliosis does not mention rotation, which is present in the most common type of scoliosis (idiopathic). The simple lateral curvature is a relatively rare finding other than in occasional nonstructural and some congenital curves. In most situations, scoliosis is a three-dimensional deformity, better described as a lordoscoliosis rather than a kyphoscoliosis. Lordosis is a curvature in the sagittal plane where the concavity is directed posteriorly. Kyphosis is the reverse. The important point in most scolioses is that there is associated vertebral rotation as well as lateral curvature of the spine. The description of a scoliosis is based on a few characteristics: the region of the curve (the site of the greatest curve angle), side of convexity (not the concavity), and Cobb angle, eg, 40° thoracic curve convex to right with the apex at T8.

Descriptive terms such as:

- major—fixed
- minor—often mobile
- primary—the initial curve or secondary (the curve generated in response to the primary curve to try to balance the spine; the compensatory curve)

are still occasionally used in relation to a double curve.

Kyphosis is an exaggeration of the normal thoracic curvature or a reversal of the normal lordotic curves in the cervical and lumbar regions. Normality is regarded as between 25–40°, with a transitional zone of 40–55°. An angle of greater than 60° is considered abnormal.

2   MEASUREMENTS

Before a management plan can be made for any patient with a deformed spine, the curve(s) must be accurately quantified. This involves assessing the size of the curve, the maturity of the patient and any underlying pathological process, eg:

- idiopathic,
- degenerative,
- tumor.

The Cobb angle [1] is the classical method for measuring the size of the curve and is defined as "the angle made by the intersection of two lines parallel to the most cranial and caudal end plate of the respective end vertebrae of a curve" (**Fig 2.3-1**). The end vertebrae are difficult to define without experience but are often those with symmetrical disc spaces and without pedicle rotation. The rib-vertebra-angle difference [3] is calculated by subtracting the angle of the rib on the convex side of the curve relative to a line perpendicular to the vertebral body endplate, from the angle on the concave side of the curve. If the rib-vertebra-angle difference < 20° and the convex rib does not overlap the vertebral body on the AP x-ray (phase I), there is a good prognosis. If the rib-vertebra-angle difference is > 20° and there is overlap between the rib and vertebral body (phase II), this gives a worse prognosis.

An assessment of skeletal maturity is made using the Risser stage [4]. This is based on the ossification of the iliac crest apophysis and is graded from 0–5; Risser 4 equates to cessation of spinal growth and Risser 5 to when the apophysis fuses to the ilium. The Risser stage relates to the potential for curve progression. If a child is young and has a low Risser stage, ie, has a lot of growth ahead of them, then there is a significant potential for worsening of an already-present curve. Conversely, if a child is older with an advanced Risser stage, then they have less opportunity for growth ahead of them, and thus less chance of curve progression. Completion of spinal growth occurs on average at 15 years 3 months in females, and 15 years 10 months in males. However, 25% of curves will continue to evolve after the full appearance of the apophysis [2]. Bone age is evaluated using an x-ray of the left wrist and hand and its comparison to the Greulich and Pyle [5] or the Tanner and Whitehouse atlas [6].

3   INVESTIGATIONS

X-rays are routinely used to confirm, quantify, and monitor progression of the deformity; note that the x-ray is a radiological test. Occasionally, CT, MRI, bone scan, and ultrasound are needed to confirm the etiology and any other associated abnormalities in other systems (**Table 2.3-1**).

MRI is used to discover any Chiari malformation, cord abnormality, eg, syrinx (**Fig 2.3-2**), diastematomyelia, or cord tethering. Some surgeons employ MRI in all preoperative scoliosis patients, while others use MRI in patients with curves at higher risk of abnormality, eg, left-sided thoracic congenital scoliosis, or patients with clinical neurological abnormalities.

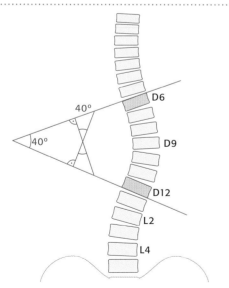

Fig 2.3-1
Method of measuring the Cobb angle.

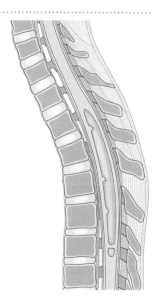

Fig 2.3-2
Thoracic syrinx.

Investigation	Reason for investigation	Problems
X-ray	Standing posteroanterior (PA) plain x-rays of entire spine to include iliac crests to assess Risser status. Side-bending PAs are useful as a preoperative investigation only for the selection of fusion levels. Lateral films are always necessary, especially if the patient has a suspected congenital scoliosis, a painful scoliosis or a sagittal plane deformity, eg, hypo or hyperkyphosis or spondylolisthesis.	The PA is used instead of AP to reduce radiation dose to breast tissue (this is very active tissue in pubertal girls and thus more susceptible to radiation exposure).
CT	3-D CT allows visualization of vertebral deformity in complex congenital abnormalities but in general is not necessary.	Exposure of patient to a large radiation dose.
MRI	An MRI study is indicated for selected cases such as patients with a congenital scoliosis, excessive kyphosis, early-onset scoliosis, left thoracic curves, or associated syndromes, with rapid progression of curve magnitude, neurological symptoms or signs, and any patient with a painful scoliosis. In this selected population, MRI demonstrates abnormalities in approximately 1/3 of cases.	MR images cannot be obtained with stainless steel implants due to gross image distortion. With titanium implants and computer software, acceptable images can be obtained. Also, stainless steel heats up in a magnetic field and is uncomfortable for the patient.
Special tests	Stagnara's plan of choice [7] is a view perpendicular to the true coronal plane of the apical vertebra. The Leeds lateral [8] is a true lateral at 90° to the plan of choice. Bone age films are necessary in selected cases.	

Table 2.3-1
Radiological investigations for spinal deformity.

4   CHILDHOOD DEFORMITY

4.1   SCOLIOSIS

Classification

Adolescent idiopathic scoliosis has been classified by Lenke [9] (**Table 2.3-2**) and King-Moe [10]. These classifications, along with the Scoliosis Research Society outcome instrument [11], can be used to evaluate the patient-based outcome of its surgical treatment. They are used in an attempt to clarify which levels need to be fused to realign the spine and maintain stability, and how useful surgery is to the patient.

The Lenke classification in idiopathic scoliosis has six main types. There are also two modifiers which are added based on the lateral view and the position of the lumbar spine on the AP x-ray. In this chapter only the six main types are addressed.

This classification is accepted by many spine surgeons as the gold standard when addressing scoliosis and it comprises three components:

- the curve type,
- the lumbar spine coronal modifiers,
- the thoracic sagittal modifiers.

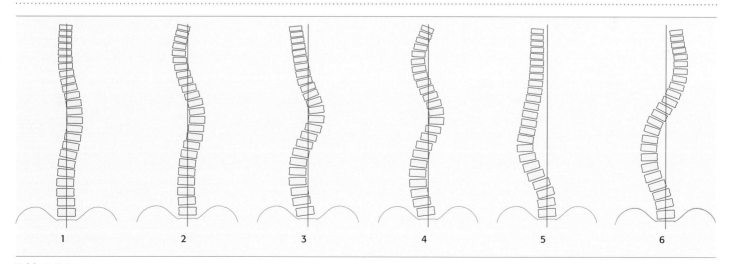

Table 2.3-2
The six main curves of the Lenke classification.

In order to determine the course of treatment and surgical management the following x-rays are required:

- standing posteroanterior x-ray,
- lateral x-ray,
- both a right and left supine bending x-ray.

Stage one of the classification involves dividing the spinal column into three regions as below:

- Proximal thoracic with the apex situated at T3, T4, or T5.
- Main thoracic with the apex between T6 and the T11/T12 disc.
- Thoracolumbar/lumbar with the apex at T12 or L1 for the thoracolumbar curves, and between the L1/L2 disc for lumbar curves.

A Cobb measurement is obtained for each, the curves are then classified as major or minor with the largest curve classed as the major one. The remaining curves are then seen as structural or nonstructural depending on the flexibility and sagittal alignment.

The three spinal regions associated with reference to sagittal angulations are the following:

- proximal thoracic (T2–5),
- main thoracic (T5–12),
- thoracolumbar/lumbar (T10–L2).

The six curve types become known when the major and minor curve patterns are combined as shown below and illustrated in **Table 2.3-2**:

- Type 1—main thoracic (MT)
- Type 2—double thoracic (DT)
- Type 3—double major (DM)
- Type 4—triple major (TM)
- Type 5—thoracolumbar/lumbar (TL/L)
- Type 6—thoracolumbar/lumbar–main thoracic (TL/L–MT)

The remainder of pediatric scolioses are divided into structural and nonstructural curves and subdivided as shown in **Table 2.3-3**.

Management

Treatment options for children with scoliosis are to watch and wait, brace, and surgery. For a skeletally immature patient (Risser 0–2), the generally accepted criteria for bracing are a curve in the range 20–45°, documented progression and acceptance for wearing a brace. The number of hours a brace should be worn is still controversial. Previously it was recommended to wear a brace for 23 hours a day, but more recently part-time bracing has been shown to also be effective. Whatever regime is used, bracing should be continued until skeletal maturity. Night-time bracing is usually proposed when the patient is at Risser 4. Surgery is indicated when there is a failure of bracing or a progressive curve greater than 40–45° in a growing child.

Nonstructural	Postural		
This is generally a mild, non-rotated scoliosis that has the potential to be fully corrected by active or passive bending and to be completely resolved after correcting the underlying cause. The cause is likely to be non spinal in origin.	**Hysterical** **Sciatic** **Inflammatory** **Compensatory**		
Structural This is a fixed deformity and there is often a rotary element. There is generally a spinal cause.	**Idiopathic** Up to 85% of structural curves. **The Lenke, King Moe, and SRS classifications only apply to the idiopathic curves.**	**Early onset** (alternative nomenclature: infantile, ie, birth to 3 years; early juvenile, ie, juvenile is classed as 4 to 10 years).	Birth to 5 years. Left thoracic curve more common (90%). More common in males. 60–70% resolve spontaneously (in this group, the scoliosis generally appears in the first 6 months of life and resolves by 2 years). Increased risk of cardiopulmonary compromise. Rib-vertebra-angle difference useful in predicting progression.
		Late onset (alternative nomenclature: late juvenile, adolescent, ie, over 10 years).	6 years and older. Right thoracic curve more common. Also there is often a thoracic hypokyphosis. More common in females (5:1). Worse prognosis if curve appears early and patient matures late, as there is more time over which the curve can progress. Curves can also progress rapidly during the adolescent growth spurt. Pulmonary function decreases in curves greater than 70° particularly with a thoracic hypokyphosis. Poor prognosis if curve greater than 45° or Rib-vertebra-angle difference greater than 20°.

Table 2.3-3
The remainder of pediatric scolioses are divided into structural and nonstructural curves and subdivided as shown here.

Structural (cont)	**Neuromuscular** Tends to be a long, C-shaped curve with a potential for pelvic obliquity and hip contractures. Major respiratory impairment is possible in this group of patients.	**Upper motor neurone**	Cerebral palsy Spinocerebellar degeneration Friedreich's ataxia Hereditary motor and sensory neuropathies Trauma Spinal tumor Syringomyelia
		Lower motor neurone	Poliomyelitis Trauma Spinal muscular atrophy I–IV (usually right-sided curve)
		Myopathies	Arthrogryposis Muscular dystrophies **Duchenne and Beckers** The incidence of a progressive scoliosis is about 95%. The curve often progresses to more than 100%. After the child begins to use a wheelchair, there is an average of 10° increase in thoracic scoliosis for each year of life. **Limb girdle** **Facioscapulohumeral** Myotonia dystrophica
	Congenital The neural axis and spinal column develop simultaneously and thus there is a risk of cord abnormalities in congenital scoliosis. An MRI scan is therefore always needed. In addition, a congenital scoliosis does not always have a major rotational component.	**Failure of information (hemivertebra)** **(Fig 2.3-3)**	**Partial unilateral** • wedge vertebra **Complete unilateral** • fully segmented (more common, more potential for curvature as two open growth plates) • semi segmented • incarcerated (least common, least potential for curve progression).

Table 2.3-3   (cont)
The remainder of pediatric scolioses are divided into structural and nonstructural curves and subdivided as shown here.

Structural (cont)	Congenital (cont)	Failure of segmentation	Partial or unilateral—a bar (more common)
			Complete or bilateral—a block
		Mixed	The worst case would be a unilateral unsegmented bar with contralateral hemivertebra
	Others		Achondroplasia
			Mesenchymal disorders, eg, Marfan syndrome (75% may have spinal involvement), Ehlers-Danlos syndrome
			Spina bifida
			Neurofibromatosis
			Rheumatoid disease
			Infection
			Spinal dysraphism

Table 2.3-3   (cont)
The remainder of pediatric scolioses are divided into structural and nonstructural curves and subdivided as shown here.

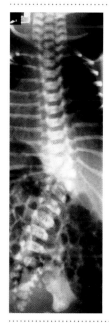

Fig 2.3-3
Right hemivertebra at thoracolumbar junction. Note sharp angulation.

In patients with muscular dystrophy, pulmonary function begins to decline rapidly when they become a wheelchair-user and can quickly get to a level where surgery is impossible. Surgery in these patients must be early and is indicated to improve quality of life and maintain the ability to sit upright in a wheelchair. It is often performed when their curves reach only 20–30° but their forced vital capacity is still greater than 40°.

The aims of surgery for scoliosis are to prevent progression of the curve, correction if possible while maintaining spine and pelvic balance, maintaining respiratory function, reducing pain, and preserving the neurological status. Cosmesis, however, is often the most important aim to the patient. Patients are often ambivalent towards the scoliosis, but any rib prominence is poorly tolerated. This can often be surgically rectified by a partial thoracoplasty, where the ribs involved in the prominence are resected and used as bone graft for the spinal fusion. The periosteum of the rib is preserved to allow the ribs to regrow in a more acceptable position.

Surgery can be posterior, anterior (via a thoracotomy, thoracoabdominal, or thoracoscopic approach), and sometimes both. The method of surgery will depend on rigidity of the curve and the number of levels to fuse. Patients requiring both anterior and posterior surgery may have fewer complications if both procedures are performed on the same day rather than separated by a 1–2 week interval. This depends on the general condition of the patient as well as the skill and speed of both surgeon and anesthetist.

Complications of surgery

Complete resolution of a large curve is almost impossible without risking significant neurological injury and so a residual curve may have to be accepted. However, a smaller curve may be returned to complete normality. If posterior fusion alone is performed in an immature child, continued anterior growth may lead to the crankshaft phenomenon where the continued anterior growth in the presence of a fused posterior spine leads to a twisting deformity.

Superficial wound infections are usually easy to treat if caught early. However, deep infection around the metalwork is very difficult to eradicate without removing the implants. Fortunately this complication is rare.

Implants have a finite life expectancy in the presence of recurrent bending and/or twisting forces. They can rapidly reach their fatigue limit and break if the bone graft does not incorporate.

Intraoperative neurological injury is unusual. However somatosensory- or motor-evoked potential (SSEP or MEP) monitoring is used with posterior surgery to reduce the risk of unavoidable neurological injury. In anterior surgery, the vertebral body is fully visualized to reduce the risk of inadvertent injury by screws. Another method of observing neurological status is the Stagnara wake-up test, which consists of waking the patient during the operation, after the correction, and asking the patient to move his legs. Obviously this is done by an experienced anesthetist in such a way that the patient does not feel any pain and doesn't remember the event.

4.2   KYPHOSIS

Classification

Kyphotic deformities are less common than scoliosis but can have serious neurological consequences due to tenting of the spinal cord. Congenital kyphosis, like congenital scoliosis, can be caused by a failure of formation or segmentation or both. Failure of formation is more common. If the failure of formation involves the anterior, or more commonly anterolateral portion of the vertebral body, then the spinal column above is pushed into an increasingly severe kyphotic deformity as growth progresses. The spinal cord (being posterior to the body) becomes more and more stretched over this deformed body. This deformity is progressive and can lead to paraplegia.

There are other causes of kyphosis such as:

• Scheuermann kyphosis
• posttraumatic fractures
• osteomalacia
• osteoporosis
• tumor collapse

Management

Treatment of a congenital, progressive kyphosis is surgical and does not involve braces or traction. The surgery can be posterior in early cases to try and achieve a convex growth arrest, or anterior and posterior in late cases where the anterior release is needed along with strut grafts to allow fusion as well as stabilization posteriorly. However, nonoperative treatment can be successful in other kyphoses.

4.3   ASSOCIATED ANOMALIES

It is important not to focus all attention on the scoliosis when radiologically assessing a patient with scoliosis or kyphosis. In some patients, the scoliosis may be a secondary phenomenon resulting from an underlying abnormality (such as in neuromuscular curves), which may predispose the patient to other problems, eg:

• renal calculi,
• recurrent renal tract infections,
• bowel problems.

In congenital scoliosis, anomalies are sometimes noted in other systems. These anomalies should be actively sought both clinically and radiologically when the congenital scoliosis is found. The etiology connecting them is unknown but is thought to be a problem of defective mesodermal development before the seventh week of embryonic growth. These anomalies are grouped under the acronym **VACTERLS:**

• **V**ertebral bars and blocks
• **A**nus
• **C**ardiac
• **T**racheal
• **E**sophageal atresia
• **R**enal
• **L**imb
• **S**ingle umbilical artery [12]

An MRI scan should be performed on these patients as well as an ultrasound of the kidneys.

4.4   NONSCOLIOSIS/NONKYPHOSIS CAUSES OF DEFORMITY

Spondylolisthesis

The word spondylolisthesis (from the Greek words spondylous = spine and olisthesis = slip) was first used by Killian in 1854 (who felt the problem was due to facet subluxation) but the pathology had been first noted in 1772 by Herbiniaux, a Belgian obstetrician, in a woman with a difficult delivery caused by obstruction of the pelvic outlet by a forward slip of the L5 on the sacrum.

Spondylolisthesis is defined as the nonanatomical alignment of one vertebra on another, most commonly anteriorly. This most frequently affects L5/S1. The slip is quantified as either low grade (anterior translation less than 50% of the horizontal length of the adjacent vertebra) or high grade (translation greater than 50%). It has also been quantified by Meyerding (**Table 2.3-4**).

Spondylolisthesis is found in up to 6% of 18-year-olds. It has a higher incidence in males, but it is more likely to progress to a high grade slip in females. Its etiology is multifactorial, related to genetic, developmental and biomechanical factors. It does have a relationship to spina bifida occulta in as much as this is related to posterior element dysplasia.

There are two commonly used classification systems for spondylolisthesis; the Wiltse, Newman, Macnab classification [14], and the Marchetti-Bartolozzi classification [15] (**Table 2.3-5**). Most cases of low-grade spondylolisthesis do not require surgery. However, those that are symptomatic or causing neural compression can be treated with fusion.

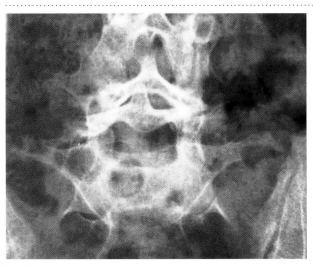

Fig 2.3-4
AP of an L5/S1 spondyloptosis (Meyerding grade V spondylolisthesis) showing the "Napoleon's hat" sign.

Grade I	up to 25% slip
Grade II	up to 50%
Grade III	up to 75%
Grade IV	up to 100%
Grade V	over 100%, ie, L5 slips off S1 anteriorly, also known as spondyloptosis [13] (**Fig 2.3-4**)

Table 2.3-4
Meyerding classification.

Wiltse, Newman, Macnab (1976)		Marchetti-Bartolozzi	
Type I	Dysplastic type due to dysplastic sacral facet	**Developmental**	High dysplastic (greater risk of high grade slip) Low dysplastic Lysis or elongation
Type II	Isthmic type with a bilateral pars lesion, either from a fatigue fracture (IIA) or from pars elongation (IIB)		
Type III	Degenerative type due to chronic instability	**Acquired**	Degenerative Traumatic (acute or stress) Pathological Postsurgery
Type IV	Traumatic due to acute fracture		
Type V	Pathological due to generalized bone disease/tumor (including spondylolisthesis acquisita or postsurgical)		

Table 2.3-5
A comparison of the classification systems for spondylolisthesis.

5   ADULT DEGENERATIVE DEFORMITY

Adult degenerative rotary scoliosis is a manifestation of severe accelerated degenerative disease of the lumbar spine. Surgery is indicated for one of two reasons: instability or neural compression. Instability usually manifests itself by mechanical pain (pain that is deep and agonizing in nature and is worsened by activity and improved by rest), while neural compression causes dermatomal or myotomal lower limb sensory or motor symptoms. Instability is often treated by fusion (anterior lumbar interbody, posterior lumbar interbody, or posterolateral fusion), with the neural compression being treated by decompression of the nerve roots at the same time.

Spinal deformity is often thought of as only-childhood scoliosis. If this were so, then this alone would represent a large, complex problem that is challenging to manage. However, spinal deformity represents the similar end result of different and varied pathologies that must be fully recognized both from their basic science (anatomy, biomechanics) as well as their clinical (instability, fusion levels, neural compression) characteristics in order to achieve a clinical outcome that is acceptable to both clinician and patient.

6   BIBLIOGRAPHY

1. **Garfin SR, Vaccaro AR** (eds) (1997) *Ortho-pedic Knowledge Update: Spine.* American Academy of Orthopedic Surgeons; 183-194.
2. **Greulich WW, Pyle SI** (1959) *Radiographic Atlas of Skeletal Development of the Hand and Wrist.* 2nd ed. Stanford: Stanford University Press; London: Oxford University Press.
3. **Haher TR, Gorup JM, Shin TM, et al** (1999) Results of the Scoliosis Research Society in-strument for evaluation of surgical outcome in adolescent idiopathic scoliosis: a multicenter study of 244 patients. *Spine;* 24(14):1435-1440.
4. **King HA, Moe JH, Bradford DS et al** (1983) The selection of fusion levels in thoracic idiopathic scoliosis. *J Bone Joint Surg Am;* 65(9):1302-1303.
5. **Lenke LG, Betz RR, Harms J et al** (2001) Ado-lescent idiopathic scoliosis: a new classifica-tion to determine extent of spinal arthrodesis. *J Bone Joint Surg Am;* 83-A:1169-1181.
6. **Lovell and Winter's pediatric orthopaedics** (1996) 4th ed. Philadelphia: Lippincott-Raven.
7. **du Peloux J, Fauchet R, Faucon B, et al** (1965) [The plan of choice for the radiologic examination of kyphoscolioses]. *Rev Chir Orthop Reparatrice Appar Mot;* 51(6):517-524.
8. **Deacon P, Flood BM, Dickson RA** (1984) Idiopathic scoliosis in three dimensions. A ra-diographic and morphometric analysis. *J Bone Joint Surg Br;* 66(4):509-512.
9. **Marchetti PG, Bartolozzi P** (1997) Spondylo-listhesis: classification of spondylolisthesis as a guideline for treatment. Bridwell, KH, Dewald RL, Hammerberg KL et al (eds) *The Textbook of Spinal Surgery.* 2nd ed. Philadelphia: Lip-pincott-Raven,1211-1254.
10. **Mehta MH** (1972) The rib-vertebra angle in the early diagnosis between resolving and pro-gressive infantile scoliosis. *J Bone Joint Surg Br;* 54(2):230-243.
11. **Meyerding HW** (1990) Spondylolisthesis and spondylolysis. Youmans JR (ed) *Neurological Surgery.* Philadelphia: WB Saunders; 2749-2784.
12. **Risser JC** (1958) The iliac apophysis, an invalu-able sign in the management of scoliosis. *Clin Orthop;* 11:111-119.
13. **Tanner JM, Whitehouse RH, Takaishi M** (1966) Standards from birth to maturity for height, weight, height velocity and weight ve-locity: British children 1965 II. *Arch Dis Child;* 41(220): 613-635.
14. **Terminology Committee of the Scoliosis Re-search Society** (1976) A Glossary of Scoliosis Terms. *Spine;* 1:57-58.
15. **Wiltse LL, Newman PH, Macnab I** (1976) Classification of spondylolysis and spondylolis-thesis. *Clin Orthop Relat Res;* 117:23-29.

2.4   THE INJURED SPINE

1   INTRODUCTION

The topic of spinal fractures and dislocations is immense. The aim of this chapter is to introduce some basic concepts and discuss the common fractures and their treatment options.

Spinal fractures and dislocations are usually the result of high-energy injuries, eg, road traffic accidents (45%) and falls (20%). A delayed or missed diagnosis is not uncommon especially in polytrauma victims and those with head injuries, unconsciousness, and intoxication. Traumatic fractures occur in a ratio of approximately four males to every female. Spinal cord injury occurs in 40–50 people per million of the population. Approximately 10–30% of patients with spinal trauma will have spinal cord injury. Of note, 5% will have deterioration in their neurology while in hospital.

The approximate percentages of all injuries occurring in the spine are:

- 55% cervical,
- 15% thoracic,
- 15% thoracolumbar,
- 15% lumbosacral.

Fractures and dislocations tend to occur at the sites of greatest movement. The thoracic spine is relatively rigid and fractures tend to be seen more commonly at the cervicothoracic and thoracolumbar junctions.

Fractures can occur with minimal trauma in patients with predisposing conditions such as osteoporosis and spinal tumor metastases. Over the age of 75 years, 60% of spinal fractures result from simple falls in the presence of underlying osteoporosis and are more common in women.

2   CLASSIFICATION AND STABILITY

There are many different types of spinal fracture and classification systems have been developed in order to standardize nomenclature, improve communication between clinicians, guide treatment, predict outcome, and give specific information such as stability of the fracture and the likelihood of neurological injury. AOSpine has developed a two-column classification of thoracic and lumbar spinal injuries (see 8.2 Thoracolumbar trauma, **Fig 2.4-9**, in this chapters). The anterior column comprises the vertebral bodies which resist compression and transmit the majority of the body's weight (a strut). The posterior column comprises the neural canal and posterior spinal elements. The majority of the body's weight lies anterior to the spine and the posterior column acts as a tension band preventing the body from falling forward, thus maintaining upright posture.

The concept of spinal stability is paramount when managing patients with vertebral injuries. Spinal stability refers to the ability of the spine under normal physiological loads to limit displacement so as to prevent injury or irritation to the spinal cord and nerve roots, and to prevent incapacitating deformity or pain due to structural changes. There are various scoring systems which help define the stability of a specific fracture.

3   EVALUATION OF SPINAL TRAUMA

The advanced trauma life support (ATLS) method is the safest way to approach trauma patients. It is systematic and addresses the major life-threatening problems in the following order:

- Airway
- Breathing
- Circulation
- Disability
- Extremities

Spinal injuries can be devastating, in particular cervical spine injuries as they can result in quadriplegia and dependence on ventilatory support (the phrenic nerve, C3, 4, 5 keeps the diaphragm alive). There is a 5–15% incidence of noncontiguous vertebral injuries, ie, those with one fracture have a 5–15% chance of having another elsewhere. Spinal injuries are therefore assumed in all trauma patients until proven otherwise. Patients have their cervical spine immobilized with a hard, rigid collar, two sandbags either side of the head, and tape placed across the forehead to secure them to the bed. This minimizes movement and potential neural damage until their cervical spine can be cleared of injury. Patients are brought into hospital on a hard spinal back board. Patients should be assumed to have unstable spinal columns until fully examined and imaged. This requires the implementation of strict precautions, eg, log rolling with cervical spine control (see chapter 3.3 Patient positioning for spine surgery).

During the ATLS primary survey for life threatening injuries, the following investigations are undertaken:

- respiratory rate,
- oxygen saturation,
- blood pressure,
- pulse,
- temperature,
- ECG,
- chest and pelvic x-rays,
- blood tests,
- the patient is often catheterized and a nasogastric tube inserted.

Arterial blood gas analysis is important in assessing the patient's respiratory function which can be affected by both chest injuries and spinal cord damage. 15% of patients with spinal trauma will have major chest injuries and 10% major abdominal injuries. The life-threatening injuries must take priority and the spinal injuries dealt with either concomitantly if safe and appropriate or at a subsequent date. Anesthetists and intensive care specialists should be involved early especially if there is evidence of cervical cord injury with subsequent respiratory compromise.

In assessing patients with spinal trauma it is vital to take an adequate medical history including the mechanism of injury. For the spine, the examination must include:

- vertebral assessment looking for posterior tenderness and deformity,
- full neurological assessment including the cranial nerves, peripheral nerves, and a rectal examination.

A formal log roll must be performed at the earliest opportunity to permit these. The hard spinal back board can then be removed. Its principle use is to protect the spine during transfer of the patient from the scene of injury to the hospital. Patients remaining on a spinal back board for prolonged periods are at a significant risk of developing pressure sores.

The control of blood pressure, oxygenation, and hematocrit is crucial to ensure adequate cord perfusion, oxygenation, and nutrition in order to prevent secondary spinal cord injury. The urine output is a good marker of global tissue perfusion.

A lateral cervical spine x-ray (showing the skull base to the C7–T1 junction) will detect up to 70–85% of abnormalities. Supplemented with AP and odontoid peg x-rays, up to 98% of injuries in the cervical spine can be identified. However, in approximately 10% of traumatic cord injuries plain x-rays will reveal no obvious evidence of bony abnormality.

The thoracic and lumbar spine are imaged using AP and lateral x-rays. Further imaging is frequently required and CT is employed to establish:

- the bony anatomy of the fracture,
- predict fracture stability,
- assess canal compromise.

While MRI can be used to look for:

- spinal cord contusion,
- hematoma,
- soft-tissue damage,
- intervertebral disc disruption.

Both modalities are often used but in general the investigation of choice depends on the type of fracture and the neurological status of the patient. CT is indicated in the majority of spinal fractures and MRI is indicated when there is:

- unexplained neurological deficit,
- incomplete neurological deficit,
- neurological deterioration,
- before reduction of a dislocation in neurologically intact patients or patients with incomplete spinal cord injuries,
- to assess ligamentous injury.

3-D CT reconstructions can be used to help in complex fractures and occasionally arteriography is employed in cervical injuries when there is vascular compromise of the vertebral arteries.

4   SPINAL AND NEUROGENIC SHOCK

Spinal shock is the period after spinal cord injury when the reflex activity of the spinal cord becomes depressed. It usually resolves within 24 hours of the injury and this is detected when the reflex arcs caudal (distal) to the injury begin to function again. The lowest of these that can be tested clinically is the bulbocavernosus reflex. This is contraction of the anus in response to bladder trigone stimulation (catheter tug) or squeezing the glans penis or tapping the mons pubis. The assessment for spinal shock is important in determining whether a patient has a complete or incomplete spinal cord injury. This cannot be determined until spinal shock has ended.

Neurogenic shock refers to the flaccid paralysis, areflexia, and lack of sensation secondary to physiologic spinal cord "shut down" in response to injury. There is reduced sympathetic outflow (T1–L2) with resultant unopposed vagal tone. There is hypotension due to loss of blood vessel tone with resultant venous pooling, and bradycardia due to reduced cardiac stimulation. This bradycardia distinguishes neurogenic shock from other types of shock, eg, hypovolemic, cardiac, and anaphylactic shock.

5   SPINAL CORD INJURY

Spinal cord injury can be primary (at the time of injury) and secondary (occurring after the injury). Primary injury can occur due to:

- contusion (bruising),
- compression (spinal canal narrowing) due to hematoma or bone which affects neuronal flow and vascularity resulting in nerve ischemia and death,
- stretch which causes vascular and axonal collapse resulting in ischemia and death,
- laceration (tear) or penetrating trauma.

Secondary injury can be due to ongoing primary injury, but it is commonly due to compromise in the blood supply to the spinal cord and edema (swelling). Spinal cord injury at the cervical level will produce quadriplegia, possible breathing problems and bladder and bowel dysfunction. At the thoracic and lumbar levels paraplegia, bladder, and bowel dysfunction result.

A complete spinal cord injury means that there is no sensation or voluntary motor function below the level of the injury. It can only be confirmed after the resolution of spinal shock when reflex activity has returned. The level of the injury is defined as the first with useful partial neurological function. This level will determine the overall functional status of the patient, eg, patients with an injury at C8 and below should be able to transfer independently, care for themselves, and use a wheelchair. The overall prognosis for recovery of neurological function in complete lesions is poor.

An incomplete spinal cord injury means that there is some function caudal to the injury. In general, the greater the function the faster the recovery and better the prognosis (but this may still take several months). Sacral sparing after spinal cord injury, ie, the presence of sacral sensation, voluntary rectal tone, and great toe movement, indicates intact long tract neurons and the potential for recovery. It is prognostic for predicting recovery except in lesions involving the conus medullaris or cauda equina. There are a variety of cord syndromes such as central, anterior, posterior, and Brown-Séquard syndrome, all of which have well-defined clinical patterns and cause incomplete spinal cord injury.

There are different classification systems used to describe spinal cord injuries but the Frankel grading is the most well known. This classifies the injury from A to E and is prognostic for recovery. Four out of five patients with spinal cord injuries will live ten or more years after the injury.

6 FRANKEL GRADING

A	Absent motor and sensory function (complete).
B	Absent motor, sensation present (incomplete).
C	Motor function present but not useful, sensation present (incomplete).
D	Motor function present and useful, sensation present (incomplete).
E	Normal motor and sensory function (normal).

Table 2.4-1
Frankel grading.

7 GENERAL MANAGEMENT PRINCIPLES

The principle aims in the management of patients with spinal trauma are to:

- preserve neurological function,
- relieve reversible nerve or cord compression,
- stabilize the spine,
- rehabilitate the patient.

There is much debate in the literature as to the indications for surgical intervention in spinal trauma. Many unstable fractures can be treated conservatively with bed rest for six or more weeks.

In general, conservative management includes:

- braces,
- molded orthoses,
- traction,
- halo jackets,
- bed rest.

Both conservative and surgical management have risks. Halo jackets in the elderly are frequently not tolerated and thus molded cervical collars are employed. The only absolute indication for surgical intervention is a nonreducible cervical facet dislocation which is causing an incomplete cord injury. In this instance it is paramount to reduce the dislocation, thereby relieving the cord compression and hopefully preventing loss of diaphragmatic function.

The other indications for surgery fall broadly under the following criteria:

- progressive neurological deficit with persistent dislocation or neurocompression not corrected by closed traction,
- persistence of incomplete spinal cord injury with continued impingement on neural elements,
- unstable dislocations that have been reduced,
- complete spinal cord injury with unstable fractures to enable early rehabilitation and aid nursing care,
- in the polytrauma setting to aid nursing and medical care,
- late instability or deformity with continued cord percussion and neurological deficit or chronic pain,
- prevent the development of or to correct posttraumatic kyphotic spinal deformity,
- unstable fractures.

Spinal fractures can be fixed by anterior, posterior, or combined surgical approaches. The anatomy of the fracture and its subsequent effects on normal spinal biomechanics and functioning must be defined prior to surgery. This allows the surgeon to plan the most suitable operation for correction. Anterior approaches are principally used to reconstruct the anterior spinal column. For example, in severe burst fractures the vertebral body can no longer support or transmit the body's weight. This makes them unstable and prone to:

- buckling forward and collapsing,
- spinal cord injury as movements can occur and fragments may retropulse into the spinal canal when weight is transmitted.

For this reason the surgeon may choose an anterior stabilization or reconstruction. Another reason for using anterior approaches is to decompress the spinal canal. For example when parts of the fractured vertebral body have retropulsed into the canal and are causing cord compression.

Posterior approaches are used to realign vertebral translation, for example in fracture dislocations. They are also used to reconstruct the posterior tension band, for example in posterior spinal column injuries. Occasionally posterior approaches can be used to decompress the spinal cord. It must be remembered that the approach and indeed indications for operation or conservative management also depends on patient factors, eg, their informed choice and their comorbidity.

Patients undergoing operations for spinal trauma must have the appropriate medical workup, which includes the tests previously mentioned. In particular, a coagulation screen and blood cross match must be performed as there can be substantial blood loss. The amount of blood cross matched will vary depending on the injury and operation. A cell saver is frequently employed to help combat this problem and prevent excessive donor blood transfusion and its associated risks. Patients can be critically unwell and difficult to intubate, especially if they have cervical trauma. The use of somatosensory-evoked potentials and motor-evoked potentials (SSEPs and MEPs) (or sometimes wake-up tests) may have a role in the neurologically intact patient when manipulation of the spinal column or deformity will occur.

The surgeon and scrub personnel must be familiar with the type of spinal instrumentation being used and the relevant kit. There are a great number of systems on the market for both anterior and posterior surgery. Pedicle screws, hooks and rods for posterior surgery can be top or side loading. Anterior surgery can include single and double adjustable rod systems as well as cages which can be fixed or expandable. When spinal fractures are stabilized they must be fused in place so that no movement can occur. In addition to the bio-inert metal instrumentation used, bone grafting is employed to allow the reconstruction to attain a biological fixation. Bone graft can be harvested locally from the fracture or from other sites such as the iliac crest. Occasionally, allograft is used from another patient, eg, femoral heads.

Surgical intervention in elderly patients is difficult because the internal fixation systems cannot adequately anchor and get secure fixation in the osteopenic bone, resulting in implant failure, eg, pedicle screw and laminar/pedicle hook pullout. In addition, elderly patients are often not medically fit to undergo major surgical procedures and the complication rates are far higher due to their comorbidity and the prolonged operative time required for a secure construct. Wound healing is reduced in these patients and bone graft less likely to take. Anterior surgery risks damage to the friable arthrosclerotic vessels (eg, aorta), and implant struts such as cages tend to fail as they cut into the soft bone. Subsequent revision surgery for implant failure to reduce pain, correct deformity, achieve stability and prevent neuronal damage carries with it a far greater morbidity and mortality as the number of instrumented levels needed to achieve this becomes greater.

8   REGIONAL INJURIES

The following is a brief synopsis of the common spinal fractures and dislocations encountered. The key to the management of spinal fractures is to prevent neurological injury, chronic pain, and deformity. Hence, the stability of any fracture must be satisfactorily determined.

8.1   CERVICAL TRAUMA

Cervical fractures represent 20–30% of all spinal fractures and objective neurological deficits or abnormalities are found in 40% of patients. Road traffic accidents cause 45% of cervical spine injuries. In patients with cervical fractures, 50% will have a fracture at an adjacent level, 15% will have a fracture elsewhere in the cervical spine, and 10% will have a fracture in the thoracolumbar spine. Because of the relatively large size of the head in relation to the body, 75% of cervical injuries in children involve the craniocervical junction. Approximately 5% of cervical spine injuries are associated with head injuries and approximately 25% of primary head injuries have cervical spine injuries. The mortality of coincident cervical spine injury and head injury is around 15%.

Cervical injuries are divided into those of C0–2 (axial) and C3–7 (subaxial). C1 and C2, the atlas and axis, are anatomically and functionally atypical vertebrae. They have distinct injury patterns with separate classifications and treatment regimes. C3–7 are the typical vertebrae and their injury patterns are classified together in a similar way to thoracolumbar fractures.

Patients with cervical spine injuries must first have their spine immobilized with a hard collar, sandbags, and tape. If there is a complete neurological deficit or deteriorating neurology with an obvious fracture dislocation of C3–7 on the plain x-ray films, traction should be applied with either a halo or Gardner-Wells tongs (see chapter 3.4 Spinal traction). If there is incomplete neurology then an MRI must first be performed to exclude a disc protrusion.

An unstable cervical spine can be predicted and defined on plain x-ray films. In general, all fractures of the occiput, atlas, and axis should be considered unstable and imaged further (CT and/or MRI). X-rays of C0–2 are often inadequate because of the overlapping facial and skull bones. An atlantodens interval (the space between the anterior arch of the atlas and the odontoid peg) which is > 3 mm in adults and > 5 mm in children is suggestive of instability.

The following suggests lower cervical spine instability:

- > 25% loss of vertebral body height,
- angular displacement of > 11° between adjacent vertebrae,
- translation of > 3.5 mm between vertebrae,
- disc space separation of > 1.7 mm.

8.1.1 C0 TO C2 FRACTURES

Occipitocervical dislocation/occipitoatlanto disarticulation
This injury is rare and is frequently due to severe high energy trauma. It is usually fatal and frequently associated with severe head trauma. Respiratory support is often needed. The immediate treatment involves in-line stabilization to attain and maintain normal alignment. Operative fixation in the form of occipitocervical instrumentation may be necessary (**Fig 2.4-1**).

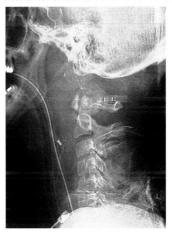

Fig 2.4-1
A lateral cervical x-ray showing an occipitocervical dislocation. The spine appears adequately aligned but there is a clear gap between C1 and the skull base. Note: the person has been intubated (an endotracheal tube is in situ).

Occipital condyle fracture

This injury occurs in compression and lateral bending and a CT scan is frequently required to make the diagnosis. The stability of the fracture is based on the degree of displacement and associated injuries. The treatment usually involves the patient wearing a rigid collar for 8 weeks. Severe unstable injuries may require a halo or surgical fusion (occipitocervical instrumentation) (**Fig 2.4-2**).

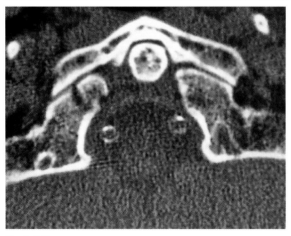

Fig 2.4-2
CT scan showing an axial cut through the skull base. The anterior arch of C1 and the odontoid peg can be seen. There is a minimally displaced fracture through the right occipital condyle. This fracture was treated conservatively in a collar.

Atlas fractures

The atlas is a closed ring and therefore fractures will occur in more than one place. Atlas fractures are often associated with odontoid peg fractures. They account for 10% of cervical spine injuries and 2% of all spinal injuries. Their stability often depends on the state of the adjacent ligaments.

A burst fracture of the atlas was first described by Jefferson in 1920. It usually occurs in axial compression, when the patient complains of an unstable neck. The patients rarely have a cord injury but vertebral artery and cranial nerve lesions can occur. Half of these fractures are associated with other cervical fractures, especially spondylolisthesis of the axis and fractures of the odontoid peg. They are usually treated in a halo jacket or rigid collar. Chronic instability or associated transverse ligament rupture is an indication for C1/2 fusion. Severe injuries may require an occipitocervical fusion (**Fig 2.4-3a–d**).

Transverse ligament ruptures are rare and usually fatal, as anterior translation of the head and atlas is unrestricted and results in a relative posterior movement of the odontoid peg causing brainstem injury. The injury normally occurs in combination with atlantoaxial subluxation or an atlas fracture. In isolated injuries, if a bony avulsion is seen there may be healing potential and a halo vest can be used to treat this injury. Otherwise a C1/2 fusion is indicated.

Atlantoaxial subluxation is another rare injury. The patient presents with the head tilted to one side. After adequate imaging, halter or halo traction and supervised exercises are usually employed. If the subluxation doesn't correct then operative reduction or a fusion in situ may be indicated.

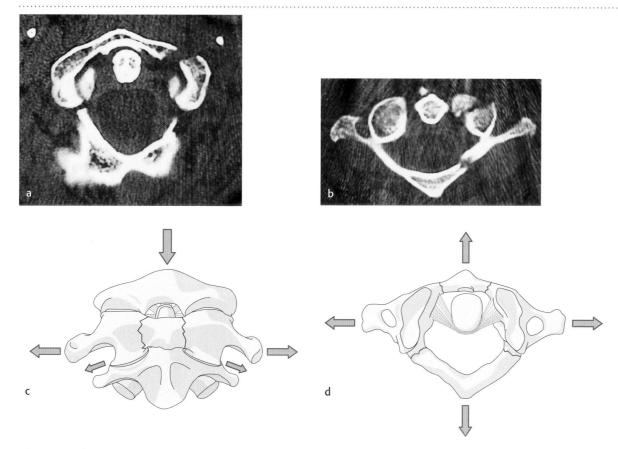

Fig 2.4-3a–d
a–b An axial CT showing a C1 Jefferson fracture.
c–d The mechanism of a Jefferson fracture.

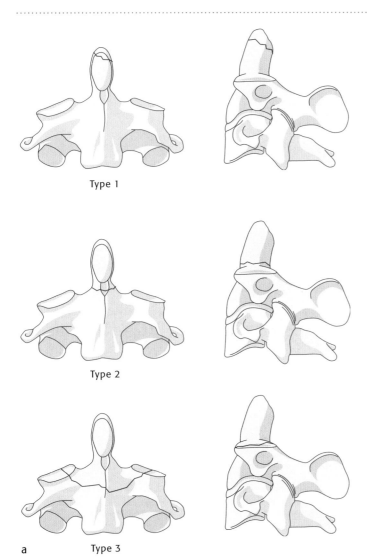

Type 1

Type 2

a   Type 3

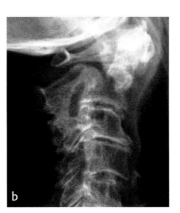

b

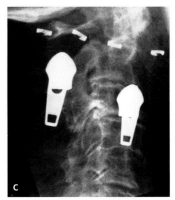

c

Fig 2.4-4a–c

a Classification of odontoid peg fractures (after Anderson and d'Alonzo).

b A lateral cervical x-ray of a type 3 peg fracture before manipulation.

c The fracture after manipulation and application of a molded collar.

Axis fractures

Odontoid peg fractures account for 10–15% of cervical spine fractures. Patients with these fractures have a 5–10% chance of neurological disturbance. Peg fractures are classified into:

- Type 1 which involves the tip (5%).
  Type 1 fractures have an intact transverse ligament, are stable, and require treatment in a collar.
- Type 2 which occurs at the junction of body and neck (65%).
  Type 2 fractures are unstable as there is nothing to stop anterior or posterior movement of the atlas on the axis and hence cord injury. They are treated in a halo jacket (or molded collar in the elderly). Reduction of displaced fractures can be performed, with the patient awake, once the halo has been applied. There is a high risk of nonunion in type 2 fractures (36%) as there is little cancellous bone. Anterior lag screw fixation or posterior C1/2 fusion may be indicated if they do not heal.
- Type 3 which extends into the body of C2 (30%).
  Type 3 fractures are treated in a similar way but are much more likely to go on to achieve union as there is plenty of cancellous bone (**Fig 2.4-4a–c**).

A hangman's fracture is a traumatic spondylolisthesis of C2 on C3 and was first described in judicial hangings. It is a fracture of the pars interarticularis of C2. They commonly occur in road traffic accidents and falls. 30% of patients will have other fractures in the cervical spine. The mechanism varies but they generally occur in hyperextension and distraction. They are classified by severity and pattern of injury. The treatment ranges from immobilization in a collar or halo jacket to open reduction followed by internal fixation by posterior and/or anterior approaches (**Fig 2.4-5a–b**).

8.1.2 C3 TO C7 FRACTURES

C3 to C7 fractures are the subaxial cervical fractures and can be classified according to the mechanism of injury (see 8.2 Thoracolumbar trauma, in this chapter).

Further imaging is paramount to assess stability and plan the treatment. Type A injuries (anterior column) are generally stable. Severe burst fractures (type A3 injuries) can be unstable as there may be significant loss of the anterior column support. It must be remembered that posterior surgery cannot provide or restore anterior column support. Anterior surgery may be indicated if the fracture is unstable and there is intervertebral disc disruption, anterior vertebral body comminution or significant canal compromise. Front and back combined approaches are used for more severe injuries. Unilateral facet

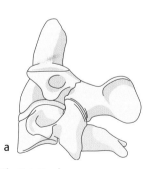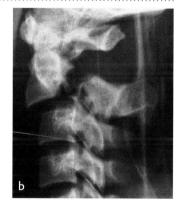

a

b

Fig 2.4-5a–b

a   A hangman's fracture

b   A lateral cervical x-ray showing a hangman's fracture. A large gap can be seen in the pars of C2 with anterior translation of the C2 vertebral body on C3.

dislocations are reduced under halo traction and sedation. Occasionally, manipulation under general anesthetic is required. This is a very dangerous procedure, because of the attendant high neurological risks. If this fails, a posterior open reduction and internal fixation is indicated provided there is no anterior disc protrusion. Bilateral facet dislocations are more unstable.

They are treated in the same way as unilateral dislocations but require operative intervention, reduction and stabilization more frequently. The clay shoveler's fracture is a stable spinous process fracture and does not usually require treatment. The shown fractures (**Fig 2.4-6a–b, Fig 2.4-7a–b, Fig 2.4-8a–b**) do require surgical intervention.

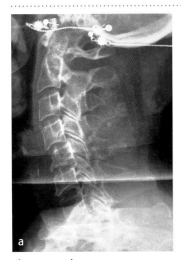 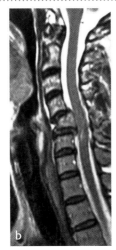

Fig 2.4-6a–b

a Lateral x-ray of the cervical spine. There is a fracture of C5 which extends through the vertebral body and posteriorly through the spinous process (both columns are involved). This is an unstable compression/flexion injury.

b The MRI shows retropulsion of the vertebral body.

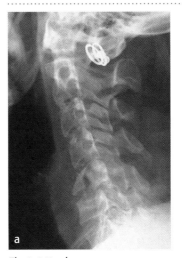 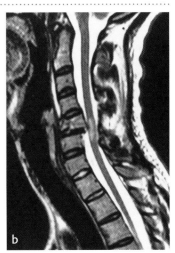

Fig 2.4-7a–b

a Lateral x-ray of a cervical spine. There is a teardrop-type fracture of the C5 vertebral body plus disruption in the alignment of the vertebral body.

b MRI shows high signal within the spinal cord and posterior soft-tissue injury.

This injury could be treated both anteriorly (spinal canal decompression and anterior column strut reconstruction) and posteriorly (restoring the posterior tension band mechanism only).

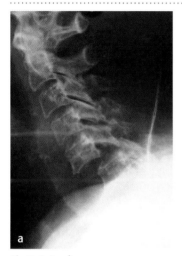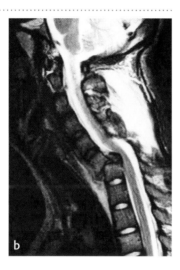

Fig 2.4-8a–b
There is a bilateral facet dislocation at C5/6 and the MRI shows a large posterior disc bulge. If this was to be reduced closed there would be a high risk of deteriorating neurology as the disc would compress the cord. This injury should be treated anteriorly by vertebrectomy and discectomy.

8.2   THORACOLUMBAR TRAUMA

The majority of thoracic and lumbar fractures occurs secondary to road traffic accidents (65%), with the incidence of neurological injury being 15–20% at the thoracolumbar level. 90% of dislocations above T10 result in complete paraplegia, while 60% below T10 result in a complete neurological deficit (the cord ends at L1/2). The thorax forms a rigid cage with the ribs attaching the spine to the sternum anteriorly. This is important because an intact nonfractured sternum and ribs will improve the stability of a fracture by acting as a strut, preventing fracture collapse and also transmitting some of the body's weight, therefore bypassing the fracture.

In the classification of thoracic and lumbar spine injuries the degree of instability and neurological deficit increases with the type of fracture. Fractures are classified into three types (A, B, C), and each type has three groups (1, 2, 3) (**Fig 2.4-9**). The classification of thoracolumbar fractures corresponds to the severity and stability of the fracture. Neurological insult occurs in approximately:

- 14% of type A,
- 32% of type B,
- 54% of type C injuries.

Minor (stable) fractures of the thoracolumbar spine tend to be isolated. They are comprised of:

- articular process fractures,
- transverse process fractures,
- spinous process fractures, and
- pars interarticularis fractures.

Once more serious fractures are excluded these minor ones are generally treated symptomatically.

Unstable fractures can be anticipated if there is a neurological deficit, clinical posterior tenderness, and/or deformity. On plain x-rays it can be predicted if there is:

- > 15–25° kyphosis,
- > 50% loss of vertebral height,
- > 50% canal compromise,
- multiple adjacent fractures,
- a scoliosis > 10°.

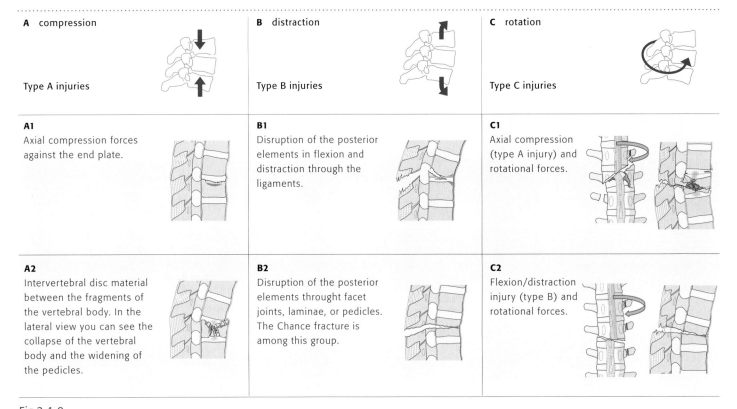

A compression

Type A injuries

B distraction

Type B injuries

C rotation

Type C injuries

A1
Axial compression forces against the end plate.

A2
Intervertebral disc material between the fragments of the vertebral body. In the lateral view you can see the collapse of the vertebral body and the widening of the pedicles.

B1
Disruption of the posterior elements in flexion and distraction through the ligaments.

B2
Disruption of the posterior elements throught facet joints, laminae, or pedicles. The Chance fracture is among this group.

C1
Axial compression (type A injury) and rotational forces.

C2
Flexion/distraction injury (type B) and rotational forces.

Fig 2.4-9
Classification of injuries in the thoracic and lumbar spine.

A3
Disruption of the posterior wall of the vertebral body and encroachment into the canal. Therefore, neurological damage is often seen.

B3
Disruption of the anterior elements in extension and retrolisthesis.

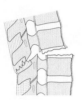

C3
Rotational and shear forces.

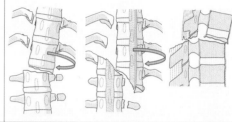

Type A injuries in general
Only the anterior column is affected in type A injuries, which focus almost exclusively on fractures of the vertebral body. Due to axial compression, the height of the vertebral body is reduced, while the posterior ligamentous complex remains intact. There are three groups for type A fractures: A1 (fractures caused by compression, not fragmentation, of the cancellous bone), A2 (split fractures in the coronal or sagittal plane with a variable degree of dislocation in the main fragments), and A3 (burst fractures in which the vertebral body is either completely or partially comminuted with centrifugal extrusion of fragments).

Type B injuries in general
Type B injuries are diagnosed based on a posterior injury and are described as transverse disruptions with elongation of the space between the posterior and anterior vertebra. The description of the mechanism involved in the lesion is used to subdivide type B injuries. Whereas B1 (posterior disruption, predominantly ligamentous) and B2 fractures (posterior disruption, predominantly osseus) are a flexion-distraction injury, B3 fractures (anterior disruption through the disc) are categorized as a hypertension-shear injury.

Type C injuries in general
Due to the rotational and shear forces that cause C type injuries, the reconstruction of the spine starts with a posterior approach in order to realign the spine. Anterior reconstructions should be considered for additional decompression or to add anterior support. Based on these factors, the alternatives discussed previously for treatment of type A and type B injuries are applicable to C1 and C2 injuries. C3 injuries are the most severe injuries of the spinal column, the majority of them being associated with paraplegia.

Fig 2.4-9 (cont)
Classification of injuries in the thoracic and lumbar spine.

In cases of unstable fractures further imaging is required and surgery may be indicated as discussed previously. The surgical approach can be anterior, posterior or both depending on the nature of the fracture and the aims of surgery. There is no clear evidence that surgery improves the neurological outcome in thoracolumbar injuries. When surgery for thoracolumbar fractures is being considered, the following goals need to be considered:

- Neurological
  – clearance of canal compromise
  – improvement of neurological deficit.
- Biomechanical
  – correction of deformity
  – stabilization of instability.

Anterior surgery should be considered if there is:

- incomplete neurological deficit,
- significant canal compromise,
- excessive vertebral body damage.

Posterior surgery should be considered if there is:

- damage to the posterior tension band,
- significant translation deformity which needs to be reduced.

Posterior spinal canal decompression in trauma risks manipulation and damage to the fragile spinal cord. The majority of neural compression occurs due to the anteriorly fractured vertebral body. Fracture dislocations with significant vertebral body disruption and translational deformity may require initial posterior surgery to reduce the deformity, with subsequent anterior surgery to clear the canal and reconstruct the anterior column support (**Fig 2.4-10a–d, Fig 2.4-11a–d, Fig 2.4-12a–d**).

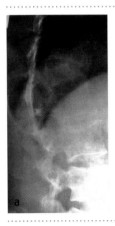 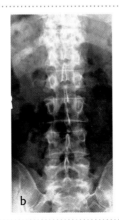 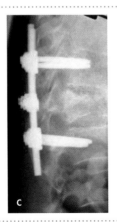 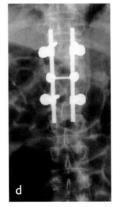

Fig 2.4-10a–d
These pre- and postoperative x-rays show a fracture dislocation of T12/L1. This was treated primarily by posterior correction.

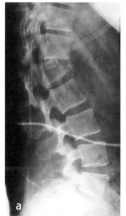 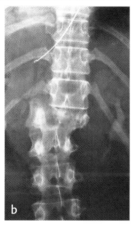 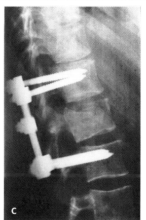 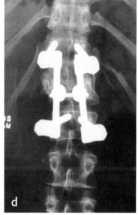

Fig 2.4-11a–d
The AP and lateral x-rays show a fracture dislocation of T12/L1. A vertebral body translation can be seen on the AP and a kyphotic deformity on the lateral x-ray. This was treated primarily by posterior correction.

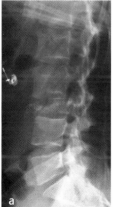 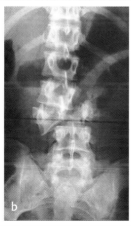 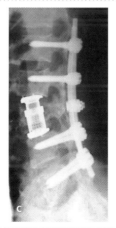 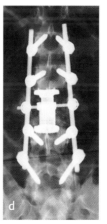

Fig 2.4-12a–d
There is a fracture dislocation of L3/4 with almost complete destruction of L3. Of note, the lateral x-ray does not fully demonstrate the severity of the injury. This illustrates the importance of taking both AP and lateral x-rays to assess fracture anatomy. This has been treated by posterior realignment and instrumentation and then anterior column reconstruction with a cage.

Chance fractures most commonly occur in the upper lumbar spine. They were first described as a pure bony injury extending from posterior to anterior. They are flexion distraction injuries and are associated with a high rate of intraabdominal injuries. They can be treated with closed reduction and extension bracing but often require surgery (**Fig 2.4-13a–b**).

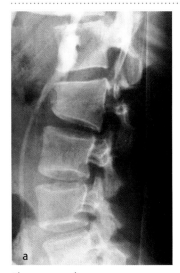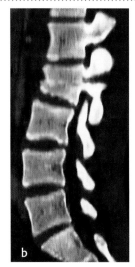

Fig 2.4-13a–b
The x-ray and sagittal CT reconstruction show an L2 bony chance fracture. This fracture extends through the body and posterior elements of L2; this was treated conservatively in a molded orthosis in extension.

8.3   SACRAL FRACTURES

Around 90% of sacral fractures are associated with pelvic trauma. These are high velocity injuries which occur in the young population. The remaining 10% are isolated low-velocity fractures which tend to occur in the elderly secondary to simple falls and minimal trauma (insufficiency fractures). There are three types of sacral fractures (**Fig 2.4-14a–c**).

- Zone 1 fractures occur in the sacral ala.
- Zone 2 through one or more of the sacral foramina.
- Zone 3 transgressing the central sacral canal.

Zone 3 injuries are the most serious, with over 50% associated with neurological injury. The management principles are the same as those discussed above. Operative fixation varies and depends on:

- the associated pelvic fracture,
- whether the sacral fracture is vertical or transverse,
- whether the lumbosacral articulation is involved.

Insufficiency (osteoporotic) fractures are generally treated conservatively.

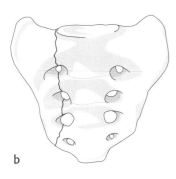

a

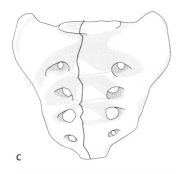

b

c

Fig 2.4-14a–c
Illustrations of the 3-zone classification of sacral fractures.
a   Zone 1.
b   Zone 2.
c   Zone 3.

9   COMPLICATIONS

The complications of spinal fractures are legion. In addition to associated injuries and spinal cord injury, as discussed above, the following are frequently encountered:

- Shock and reduced end organ perfusion, eg, low blood pressure causing renal failure.
- Pain secondary to the fracture.
- Urinary infections secondary to bed rest or indwelling catheters.
- Chest infections secondary to bed rest or respiratory dysfunction in cervical injuries.
- Ileus and large bowel pseudobstruction. This is dysfunction of the large and or small bowel which can occur secondary to neurological injury, immobility and spinal and pelvic fractures.
- Gastric stress ulcers, bleeding and perforation secondary to the body's stress response and reduced gastric perfusion.
- Thromboembolism (deep venous thrombosis and pulmonary embolus) due to immobility. Adequate fluid hydration and thromboembolic deterrent (TED) stockings, flowtron boots or arterial venous (AV) foot pumps should be used to prevent this. Chemical thromboprophylaxis with anticoagulants (eg, heparin) should always be considered. This should not be given perioperatively because of the risk of epidural bleeding and cord compression.
- Pressure sores due to immobility, especially the heels, sacrum and buttocks. These can be devastating and patients on bed rest should be log rolled regularly (every two hours). It is also important to check the skin behind braces and collars.

- Autonomic dysreflexia. This is a generalized sympathetic discharge resulting in headache, nausea, chills, anxiety, sweating, and hypertension.
- Depression.

Operative complications include:

- blood loss and transfusion,
- nerve and spinal cord injury,
- implant failure either during the operation or subsequently,
- failure of fusion, nonunion and pseudarthrosis (a false joint),
- infection and wound problems,
- dural tear and cerebrospinal fluid leak,
- death.

10   POSTOPERATIVE TREATMENT

It is important to manage patients with spinal injuries, especially those with spinal cord injuries, using a multidisciplinary approach. They should be treated in specialist units offering expert services including nursing staff, physiotherapists, occupational therapists, social workers, psychologists, and orthotists, all of whom are trained to look after patients with spinal injuries. Rehabilitation of the patient so that they can achieve the best possible useful outcome and come to terms with their injury and or disability is the key.

Patients who have had fractures with no neurological injury should be given realistic advice as to what they can and cannot do following discharge. They should be seen regularly in clinic to monitor their recovery and to identify and manage complications early, should they occur. Patients with neurological injuries are frequently transferred to specialist rehabilitation units. They may go on to have further nerve and bladder tests, nerve stimulators, and possibly even muscle and tendon transfer operations to help improve their functional outcome.

In the future there will be more minimally invasive surgical techniques developed, computer-assisted surgery and interventional radiology techniques. Medical interventions are being developed which will prevent spinal cord edema and ischemia secondary to trauma. In the not too distant future, nerve regeneration therapies, nerve grafting, and transplantation may become available, giving hope to those with devastating disabilities.

11   SUGGESTIONS FOR FURTHER READING

Aebi M, Thalgott JS, Webb JK (eds) (1998) *AO ASIF Principles in Spine Surgery.* 1st ed. New York: Springer-Verlag.

Devlin VJ (ed) (2003) *Spine Secrets.* 1st ed. Philadelphia: Hanley and Belfus Inc.

Koval KJ, Zuckerman JD (eds) (2001) *Handbook of Fractures.* 2nd ed. USA: Lippincott, Williams and Wilkins.

Timothy J, et al (2004) Mini-Symposium: Spinal Trauma. *Current Orthopaedics* (Elsevier); 18:1–48.

Vaccaro, AR, et al (2003) Selected Instructional Course Lectures. The American Academy of Orthopaedic Surgeons: Diagnosis and management of thoracolumbar spine fractures. *The American Journal of Bone and Joint Surgery;* 85: 2455–2470.

2   PATHOLOGY OF THE SPINE

2.5   PRIMARY AND METASTATIC TUMORS OF THE SPINE

1   INTRODUCTION

The most common neoplastic conditions affecting the spine are skeletal metastases arising from carcinomas and lympho-proliferative diseases (lymphoma and myeloma). 60% of spinal metastases are secondary to breast, lung, or prostate carcinomas [1]. There are multiple hypotheses as to the reason for this high frequency; however, the pathogenesis is still not fully understood.

At autopsy, as many as 90% of patients who die of cancer may exhibit spinal metastatic disease. Of all patients who die with metastatic carcinoma, as little as half will have symptoms from that lesion. Fewer than 10% of patients with symptomatic spinal metastases are treated surgically. With the increasing knowledge of the pathways of pain production, spinal instability, improvement of spinal instrumentation, and the longer survival of patients with spinal metastasis, a larger percentage of patients may benefit from surgical intervention.

The most common location for metastatic spinal disease is the thoracolumbar region, which accounts for 70% of all lesions. The lumbar and sacral spine account for only 20% with the cervical spine representing 10%. Some authors suggest a higher percentage occurs in the cervical spine [2]. Spinal cord compression varies with the volume of the spinal canal; this is seen more often earlier in the thoracic spine.

Primary bone tumors are rare, accounting for 0.4% of all tumors and representing only 4.2% of the primary spinal tumors. There is a larger incidence in the sacrum and cervical spine as opposed to the lumbar and thoracic spine.

The initial clinical characteristics of a patient with a spinal malignancy can vary considerably. Tumors may appear as incidental findings on x-rays or on clinical examination. Symptoms can range from mild pain, scoliosis, and stiffness to significant neurological deficits. Severe night pain is a common symptom of a malignant process.

2   EVALUATION

Pain is the most common presenting complaint for patients with spinal malignancy, which has a gradual onset and becomes progressively worse. It can be unrelenting and nonmechanical, becoming worse at night. Early on, the pain is axial but as it progresses it can become radicular as neural compression occurs.

Pathological fracture should be considered when patients complain of an acute onset of pain in the absence of a clear history of significant trauma. Neurological symptoms usually occur late in the disease process and lead to medical referral. Motor weakness and even paralysis are common presenting symptoms; numbness and paresthesias are less common presentations.

Radicular pain can accurately localize the tumor level within a few vertebral levels. It is uncommon to see isolated bowel and bladder dysfunction but when present necessitate further assessment with magnetic resonance imaging (MRI) to identify neural compression. Patients who present with progressive neurological deterioration need urgent assessment but severe deficits and rapidly progressive deficits have a much more guarded prognosis.

Other salient features in the history are:

- unintended weight loss,
- fatigue,
- anorexia,
- hemoptysis,
- hematuria,
- melena,
- hematemesis,
- smoking.

A previous history or a family history of malignancy is also important as patients with, for example breast carcinoma, may have a disease-free interval of 10–20 years.

3   PHYSICAL EXAMINATION

A general examination including a rectal examination is required, as well as a full neurological assessment. The examination should focus on areas where primary lesions commonly arise, including the prostate, chest, breasts, abdomen, and lymphatic system. Localized spinal tenderness is investigated as it can lead to the site of pathology. Multilevel tenderness may represent multilevel disease [3].

4   IMAGING

The imaging of choice in the assessment of spinal tumors includes plain x-ray, bone scans, CT scans, MRI scans, and angiography. Each modality has its advantages and disadvantages and usually plain x-ray is combined with MRI scanning.

Plain x-rays demonstrate overall spinal alignment and instability. Plain x-rays will identify 80% of benign bone tumors involving the spine as well as a significant proportion of primary or metastatic lesions. Early metastatic lesions will not be detected, as destruction of 30–50% of trabecular bone is required before a radiological abnormality is seen.

Primary bone tumors such as chondrosarcoma or osteosarcoma are usually associated with a radiodense mass extending beyond the vertebral body. Metastatic lesions may be osteolytic, osteoblastic, or mixed. Prostate and breast often produce a blastic or mixed response, whereas renal carcinoma most often is associated with a lytic response. Metastatic disease usually involves the vertebral body and is seen there seven times more frequently than in the posterior elements. Destruction of the pedicle can be seen on the AP x-ray in several cases. Lesions involving the posterior elements, especially in the younger age group, are normally benign.

Defining spinal stability using plain x-ray is controversial, but losses of 50% of vertebral height or increasing kyphosis have been recommended as useful parameters.

A technetium-99 bone scan is a useful test for screening patients with known malignancy. Bone scans can identify metastases 3–12 months before plain x-rays can detect them.

Patients with:

- lung carcinomas,
- breast carcinomas,
- prostate carcinomas,
- kidney carcinomas, or
- thyroid carcinomas.

should undergo bone scanning as part of their initial staging studies. It can detect lesions with an osteoblastic response. Unfortunately, false-negative scans do occur, commonly in tumors with little osteoblastic activity such as in multiple myeloma.

To improve specificity, single positron emission computed tomography (SPECT) has been used to localize bony activity in the vertebral body. The sensitivity and specificity of SPECT in identification of vertebral metastases are 87% and 91% respectively.

CT scans demonstrate bony integrity in benign and malignant tumors and are useful in the assessment of instability. They are also important in preoperative planning and in localization of some benign tumors, eg, osteoid osteoma. CT scans also assess pathological fractures for canal compromise and osseous impingement of the spinal cord.

MRI scanning is the imaging of choice for the evaluation of metastatic and primary diseases of the spine. It can assess bony involvement and soft-tissue extension as well as neural compression. With the sagittal images the whole spine can be assessed for potential further involvement.

It is well recognized that 10% of patients with spinal cord compression will have multiple levels of compression, and that many will also have additional vertebral involvement. Li and Poon [4] reported 93% sensitivity and 97% specificity for MRI in the assessment of metastatic disease. The differentiation of tumor from infection can be made using MRI as vertebral osteomyelitis is located adjacent to the end plates and often into the disc which is not affected with metastasis.

Angiography may be used as a diagnostic tool to demonstrate the vascularity of a tumor but it can also be used to perform preoperative embolisation of very vascular metastatic tumors such as renal carcinoma, as well as before resection of some primary tumors.

5   BIOPSY

In the preoperative workup, it is necessary to stage and diagnose the disease, evaluate the local and systemic extent of the lesion, and plan a surgical procedure where indicated. In the case of multifocal lesions, a biopsy specimen should be obtained from the most accessible lesion. There are three types of biopsy techniques available to the surgeon for a suspected lesion.

These include:

- percutaneous needle biopsy—fine-needle aspiration or a large bore under radiographic guidance,
- open incisional biopsy,
- excisional biopsy.

An excisional biopsy may be indicated for certain posterior lesions in which the differential diagnosis is limited (osteoid osteoma or osteoblastoma) [2].

The biopsy, although technically simple, is an inherently difficult procedure with a high rate of complications, some of which will materially change the course of treatment and treatment outcome. Thus, the decision on who should perform the biopsy is as critical as how it is performed. Often the referring physician either does not consider the possibility of a malignant tumor or finds the temptation to perform the biopsy difficult to resist.

When malignancy is not suspected, the evaluation is incomplete, the staging inadequate, and the procedure is improperly performed, therefore making the situation worse.

Complications in the biopsy process are much more likely to occur when the procedure is performed outside of treatment centers. Thus, if the clinical and radiographic information favors a diagnosis of malignant or aggressive benign bone tumor, the clinician should strongly consider referring to an experienced surgical oncologist without performing an invasive procedure. The surgeon performing the definitive procedure should also be involved in the staging and biopsy of the lesion.

In instances in which metastatic disease is likely, given the patient's age, location of the lesion, and medical history, a biopsy is still the last process in the staging of the disease. Routine laboratory analyses are requested, including a serum calcium and prostatic specific antigen.

Plain x-rays of the chest are mandatory to search for a primary lesion and to identify other metastatic lesions. CT scanning of the chest, abdomen, and pelvis will form part of the staging procedure, as well as a mammogram in women in which the primary lesion remains unknown.

The biopsy is then made from the most accessible lesion and with this diagnostic protocol, up to 85% of the primary sites of origin of the lesion can be identified. This protocol can occasionally negate the need for a biopsy if the above investigations make the diagnosis, such as multiple myeloma.

6   STAGING

Surgical staging is appropriate after the diagnosis has been confirmed and the staging investigations performed. The Weinstein Boriani Biagini (WBB) system was proposed in recognition of the differences between spinal and long bone tumors.

The unique vertebral anatomy and the difficulties in surgical resection require specific anatomic compartments to be delineated and the extent of the tumor to be described [5]. This system was originally proposed by Weinstein and was subsequently modified and tested.

With reference to tumor extent, the system allows for more uniform data collection so that surgical decisions can be made and multicenter studies performed. The description of the WBB staging system begins in the transverse plane where the vertebra is divided into 12 zones, starting on the left half of the spinous process (**Fig 2.5-1**). This emphasizes limitations in performing en bloc excisions because of the presence of the spinal cord. The longitudinal extent of the tumor is related to the number of segments involved. The success of surgical resection is dependent on the staging system and is related to preoperative planning and the ability to carry out the resection correctly [5].

The Enneking [6] staging system for benign and malignant primary bone tumors has been used for many years. Malignant tumors are staged according to histological grade, intra- or extracompartmental extent of the tumor and the presence or absence of metastasis.

Benign tumors are classified numerically (1–3). The stages describe the characteristics of the tumor:

A   Extraosseus soft tissues
B   Intraosseus (superficial)
C   Intraosseus (deep)
D   Extraosseus (extradural)
E   Extraosseus (intradural)

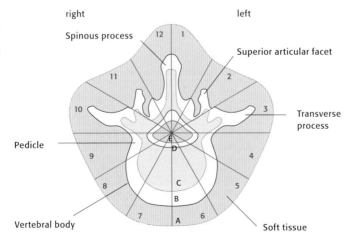

right   left

Spinous process
Superior articular facet
Transverse process
Pedicle
Vertebral body
Soft tissue

Fig 2.5-1
WBB surgical staging system. The transverse extension of the vertebral tumor is described with reference to 12 radiating zones (numbered 1 to 12 in a clockwise order) and to five concentric layers (A to E, from the paravertebral extraosseous compartments to the dural involvement). The longitudinal extent of the tumor is recorded according to the levels involved.

- Stage 1 tumors remain stable and are intracompartmental, in the vertebra.
- Stage 2 tumors have progressive growth that is limited by natural barriers such as the vertebra.
- Stage 3 tumors are aggressive and destroy barriers, showing cortical destruction and extravertebral extension.

Malignant tumors are also subdivided using roman numerals into three stages but are also subclassified into A and B, describing whether the tumor is intra- (A) or extracompartmental (B). Stage 1 tumors are low grade and stage 2 tumors high grade, whereas stage 3 tumors do not have any grade but have local or regional metastases.

Tokuhashi [7] developed a classification system to determine the prognosis and life expectancy of patients with metastatic disease. The system awards a point value to six parameters that are totaled to determine the overall prognostic score. Treatment recommendations are then related to the score.

The six parameters are:

- General health condition (poor, 0 points; moderate, 1 point; good, 2 points).
- Number of extraspinal bone metastases (≥ 3, 0 points; 1–2, 1 point; 0, 2 points).
- Number of vertebral metastases (≥ 3, 0 points; 2, 1 point; 1, 2 points).
- Metastases to major internal organs (unremovable, 0 points; removable, 1 point; no metastases, 2 points).
- Primary site of lesion (lung, stomach, 0 points; kidney, liver, uterus, others, unidentified, 1 point; thyroid, prostate, breast, rectum, 2 points).
- Spinal cord palsy (complete, 0 points; incomplete, 1 point; none, 2 points).

Patients with a total score of 9 or higher survived an average of 12 months or more, those with 8 points or fewer survived less than 12 months and those with 5 points or fewer survived less than 3 months. Therefore it was recommended that patients with a score of 9 points or greater should have an excisional procedure, whereas a palliative procedure was indicated for a patient with 5 points or fewer. No firm recommendations were made for patients with a score of 6 to 8.

Tomita [8] developed a prognostic scoring system similar to the Tokuhashi scheme to provide a treatment strategy for patients with spinal metastases. A surgical approach is determined based on a score derived from three prognostic factors.

The three factors are:

- Grade of malignancy (slow growing, 1 point; moderate growing, 2 points; rapid growth, 4 points).
- Visceral metastases (no metastasis, 0 points; treatable, 2 points; untreatable, 4 points).
- Bony metastases (solitary or isolated, 1 point; multiple, 2 points).

Summation of these three factors gives a prognostic score between 2 and 10 points. For a patient with a score of 2 to 3 points, the treatment is long-term local control with a wide or marginal excision. For a score of 4 to 5 points, marginal or intralesional excision is recommended for middle-term local control. For a score of 6 to 7 points, the treatment goal is short-term palliation. A score of 8 to 10 points indicates conservative nonoperative care.

7   BENIGN PRIMARY TUMORS

The most common benign tumors are:

- osteoid osteoma,
- osteoblastoma,
- osteochondroma,
- giant cell tumor,
- hemangioma,
- Langerhan's cell histiocytosis (previously called eosinophilic granuloma),
- aneurismal bone cysts,
- neurofibroma.

Benign primary tumors are less common than malignant primary ones. The patient's age and the location of the tumor are important prognostic indicators. Above the age of 21 years most tumors are malignant. Tumors in the posterior elements tend to be benign, whereas anterior ones tend to be malignant. Some benign tumors have an increased local recurrence rate (giant cell tumor, aneurismal bone cysts, and osteochondroma) or can be locally destructive.

Osteochondromas of the spine generally arise from the posterior elements and are rarely associated with neural compromise. Persistently painful lesions or ones producing neural symptoms can be excised. The cartilage cap needs to be excised to prevent recurrence.

Osteoid osteomas are the commonest benign vertebral tumor. They occur in teenagers and young adults and occur in the pedicles, transverse processes, and facet joint. A painful scoliosis or night pain relieved by anti-inflammatory medication suggests the diagnosis. The lesion tends to occur in the apex of the concavity of the curve. The lesion usually spontaneously resolves but surgical excision occasionally is required. Intralesional excision of the nidus is all that is necessary.

Osteoblastomas are similar to osteoid osteomas but are larger (greater than 2 cm) and anti-inflammatory medication does not relieve the pain. They have a larger soft-tissue component. The spine accounts for 40% of all cases. Intralesional or marginal excision is adequate for stage 2 lesions but marginal excision is required for stage 3 lesions with adjuvant radiotherapy.

Hemangiomas are normally detected as an incidental finding (**Fig 2.5-2a–b**). Autopsy studies have demonstrated approximately 10% of the population have asymptomatic hemangiomas in the spine. Occasionally they cause pathological fractures or cord compression, and may require surgery (**Fig 2.5-2c–d**). The vertical-orientated trabeculae seen on plain x-ray without vertebral enlargement is known as corduroy cloth appearance. If they cause pain or neural compromise they can be embolised. In most cases hemangiomas require no treatment.

Aneurismal bone cysts occur anywhere but most commonly in the thoracolumbar area and in the posterior elements. The majority occur before the age of 20 years. Aneurismal bone cysts produce cortical expansion with osteolysis. Within the central lytic area septations may give a soap bubble appearance. MRI may reveal fluid levels within the lesion. Treatment includes curettage, wide local excision, embolisation and radiation. Recurrence rates of up to 25% have been recognized.

Giant cell tumors are seen in the third and fourth decade. They occur at any level and in either anterior or posterior column. They can be locally aggressive and can metastasize. Surgical treatment usually involves extended intralesional curettage or in selected cases a marginal en bloc resection. Recurrence rates of up to 50% have been seen. Radiotherapy is indicated as adjuvant therapy in nonresectable lesions.

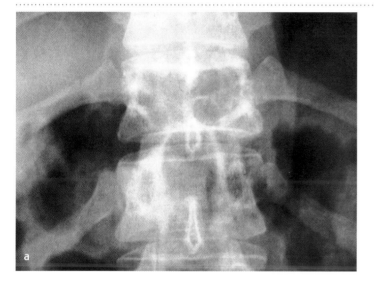

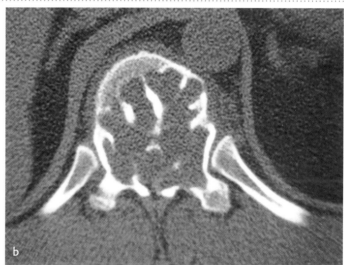

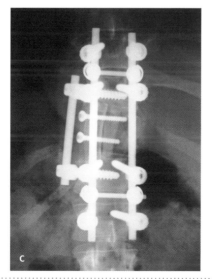

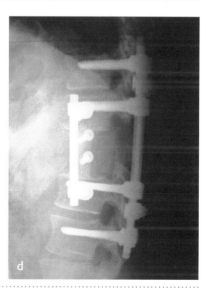

Fig 2.5-2a–d
a   AP x-ray of hemangioma at T12 preoperative.
b   MRI of hemangioma.
c–d Postoperative x-rays.
(Reproduced with kind permission of BJC Freeman.)

Langerhan's cell histiocytosis is seen in the first and second decades of life. It occurs in the vertebral body and classically appears as vertebra plana. The mainstay of treatment is observation, as the lesion is self-limiting. Bracing can be used to prevent kyphosis as the vertebra reconstitutes. Occasionally, a biopsy is required for diagnosis and curettage and low-dose radiotherapy given.

Neurofibromas arise from the nerve root or sheath. They tend to be dumbbell-shaped through the foramen with an intradural and an extradural component. Scoliosis can result. Neurofibromas need early therapy. Malignant change occurs in up to 20% of cases, especially in neurofibromatosis. Symptomatic lesions should have an en bloc resection. Otherwise, the nerve root should be preserved.

8   MALIGNANT PRIMARY TUMORS

There are three types of sarcomas affecting the spine. These are osteosarcoma, Ewing's sarcoma, and chondrosarcoma. The first two are more common in young adults, whereas chondrosarcoma is seen in the age group from 30–70 years (**Fig 2.5-3a–c**).

Ewing's sarcoma commonly occurs between the ages of 5–20 years. It can be mistaken for infection, and 5% occur in the spine. The vertebra appears moth-eaten with preservation of the discs. Treatment involves a multimodal regime of preoperative chemotherapy followed by an en-bloc resection of the vertebra with or without postoperative radiotherapy.

Osteosarcomas are uncommon in the spine and they are seen either in the second or third decades, or later in the sixth decade. The later peak usually occurs with the presence of Paget disease. The current treatment regimen is multiagent chemotherapy followed by resection of the tumor, followed again by further chemotherapy. If the tumor specimen demonstrates

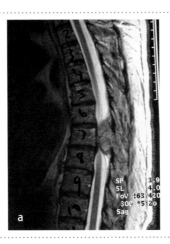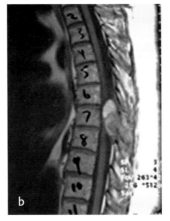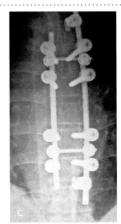

Fig 2.5-3a–c
Liposarcoma seen at T7 causing cord compression with resulting myelopathy.
a–b   Preoperative MRIs.
c   Postoperative x-ray.

9   METASTATIC TUMORS

90% tumor kill then there is a 5 year survival rate of 85%; if there is less than 90% then the survival rate is 25%

Chondrosarcomas occur more frequently than other sarcomas. They are neither chemosensitive nor radiosensitive. Therefore, the primary modality of treatment is surgical resection.

Chordomas are malignant tumors of notochordal origin arising in the vertebra. They arise strictly in the axial skeleton. They occur in the fifth to seventh decade commonly. Most (60%) occur in the sacrum, with 25% occurring in the clivus and the remainder in the cervical, thoracic and lumbar spine. They tend to be central and usually in S3 and below. They present with pain (coccydynia), constipation, and alteration in bowel and bladder function. They appear lytic on plain x-rays. MRI scans are the most effective imaging modality. Treatment is predominantly surgical as they are chemoresistant and can metastasize to both lung and bone.

The commonest tumor of the spine is a metastasis. The goals of treatment are to control pain, restore neural functioning, restore spinal stability, and prevent pathological fracture. How this is achieved is dependent on histology of the tumor, the extent of spinal involvement, other metastatic disease, sensitivity of the primary lesion, and the patient's life expectancy.

Patients present with spinal metastases in one of three ways:

- an incidental finding during a routine examination,
- in a follow-up examination as a result of a symptomatic back lesion, or
- after seeking medical advice following a neurological deficit.

Treatment is based on the life expectancy of the patient and on the classification systems mentioned above. The first line of treatment for spinal pain is radiotherapy, with chemotherapy added for tumors such as lymphoma, myeloma (**Fig 2.5-4a–c**),

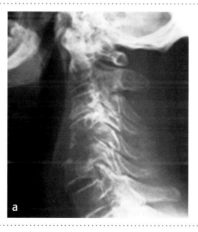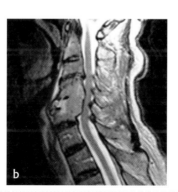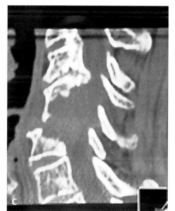

Fig 2.5-4a–c
Myeloma at C4–6 causing radicular pain, myelopathy, and spinal instability.
a X-ray.
b MRI.
c CT.

and breast and prostate carcinoma. If neural compression without neurological deficit is the source of pain then radiotherapy is advocated for a radiosensitive tumor, otherwise surgery is considered. Pain from gross instability or pathological fracture does not respond as well to radiotherapy and early surgery may be required.

A new treatment option for patients with a pathological fracture is vertebroplasty. This technique is effective for patients with mechanical pain. The vertebral body is percutaneously stabilized with a uni- or bipedicular injection of methylmethacrylate. Short-term results are encouraging.

For patients with neurological deficit an MRI scan assessment is necessary as 10% will have compression at a second area (**Fig 2.5-5a–b**). The rate of onset of the deficit has a significant effect on the prognosis. The slower progressive deterioration has a better prognosis than a more rapid onset of neurological deficit. The site of compression is anterior in 70%, lateral in 20%, and posterior in 10%. Generally, anterior decompression will be superior for an anterior tumor. Neurological recovery is better following an anterior approach as opposed to a posterior laminectomy, but a transpedicular or costotransversectomy approach with stabilization can give an equivalent decompression to that from an anterior approach with equal neurological recovery.

In the majority of cases a posterior approach is performed with stabilization using a pedicular system. Occasionally, an anterior approach is undertaken and the anterior column can be reconstructed with either cages, methylmethacrylate cement, or strut graft supplemented with a rod or plate system.

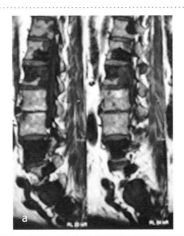 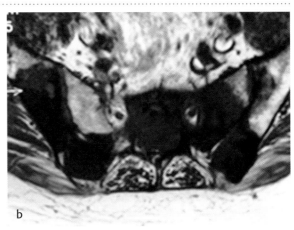

Fig 2.5-5a–b
MRI scans showing multiple metastases in the lumbar and sacral spine with compression of the cauda equina from a renal carcinoma.

Spinal neoplasms need to be divided into primary benign tumors, primary malignant tumors, and metastatic tumors. Goals of treatment must be clearly delineated and the oncologic principles for effective tumor treatment must be merged with the emerging techniques in spine surgery.

It is understood that wide resection of the neoplasm in the spine can be difficult to achieve, however, negative margins can be obtained in isolated anterior or posterior lesions. A negative margin is critical for the long-term survival of patients with chondrosarcoma, osteosarcoma, and chordoma.

Positive margins may require further adjuvant therapy. Metastatic disease of the spine has a wide clinical spectrum. When considering the appropriate treatment, not only are manifestations of the disease important, but also the patients' general condition, as well as the survival, histological type, and response to adjuvant therapy. In the treatment of these patients, techniques that require prolonged immobilization should be avoided with early mobilization and return of function the primary goal.

10   BIBLIOGRAPHY

1. **McLain RF, Weinstein JN** (1990) Tumors of the spine. *Semin Spine Surg;* 2:157–180.
2. **Abdu WA, Provencher Lt M** (1998) Primary bone and metastatic tumors of the cervical spine. *Spine;* 23(24):2767–2776.
3. **O'Connor MI, Currier BL** (1992) Metastatic disease of the spine. *Orthopaedics;* 15(5):611–620.
4. **Li KC, Poon PY** (1988) Sensitivity and specificity of MRI in detecting malignant spinal cord compression and in distinguishing malignant from benign compression fractures of vertebrae. *Magn Reson Imaging* 6(5):547–556.
5. **Boriani S, Weinstein JN, Biagini R** (1997) Primary bone tumors of the spine: terminology and surgical staging. Spine; 22(9):1036–1044.
6. **Enneking WF** (1983) *Musculoskeletal Tumour Surgery.* New York: Churchill Livingstone, 69–122.
7. **Tokuhashi Y, Matsuzaki H, Toriyama S,** et al (1990) Scoring system for the preoperative evaluation of metastatic spine tumor prognosis. *Spine;* 15(11):1110–1113.
8. **Tomita K, Kawahara N, Kobayashi T,** et al (2001) Surgical strategy for spinal metastases. *Spine;* 26(3):298–306.

2   PATHOLOGY OF THE SPINE

2.6   INFECTIONS OF THE SPINE

1   INTRODUCTION

Infections of the spine have occurred for thousands of years. Deformity from presumed spinal infection has been found in Egyptian mummies from around 3000 BC [1]. Percival Pott in 1779 reported the natural history of tuberculous spondylitis and hence, tuberculosis of the spine was named Pott disease.

It was not until Breschet [2] described the venous system of the spine in 1819 and Rodet [3] injected *Staphylococcus aureus* bacteria into the veins of animals that understanding of the blood-borne spread of vertebral osteomyelitis improved.

From postoperative wound infections to exotic bacterial infections found in intravenous drug users, spinal infections present a wide spectrum of problems for the treating clinician. Any element of the spine can be affected by invading organisms, in isolation or more commonly, in combination. Prior to the use of antibiotics, mortality approached 70%.

Spinal infections usually present with back pain and often with an absence of constitutional upset [3]. Early diagnosis is essential; hence, clinicians must have a high index of suspicion, supported by appropriate radiological and laboratory investigations, in order to obtain an optimal outcome for the patient. The aims of treating spinal infections are swift diagnosis, with isolation of the causative organism, preservation of neurological function and eradication of the infection. A stable and pain-free spine is the optimal end result for the patient.

2   EPIDEMIOLOGY

Spinal infections can be classified by:

• route of infection,
• anatomical site,
• causative organism.

3   ROUTE OF INFECTION

Infections of the spine can result from the hematogenous spread of bacteria from distant sites, most commonly from the genitourinary tract. The bacteria were once thought to reach the spine via Batson's valueless venous plexus, in an identical manner to metastases. However, this is now thought to be unlikely [4].

Alternatively, they may reach the vertebral column by local spread from adjacent tissues that have become infected. Finally, and probably the most common cause in western medical practice, is direct inoculation, be it traumatic or more often iatrogenic, for example, during spinal procedures such as discography.

4   ANATOMICAL SITE

The vertebral end plate is the most common site of infection, followed by the disc space, and finally the epidural and paraspinal regions. **Table 2.6-1** divides the spine into distinct anatomical zones that can become infected. Different organisms have preference for certain anatomical sites, eg, staphylococci in the disc and tubercle bacillus in the vertebral body.

Vertebral osteomyelitis accounts for up to 4% of all osteomyelitic infections. Males are more frequently affected than females and adults more frequently than children. The peak ages for these infections are from 45–65-years-old.

Disc space infections most commonly occur after surgical interventions. The reported incidence of postdiscectomy disc space infections ranges from 1 to 2.8%, and about 1% for discography.

Epidural abscesses are found in association with vertebral osteomyelitis in just fewer than 50%. Such an infection can spread into the meninges subdural space, or even the spinal cord.

Anatomical location	Structures involved	Clinical description
Anterior spine	Vertebral body	Vertebral osteomyelitis
		Spondylodiscitis
		Spondylitis
	Intervertebral disc	Discitis
	Paravertebral space	Paravertebral abscess
Posterior spine	Subcutaneous space	Superficial wound infection
		Infected seroma
	Subfascial space	Deep wound infection
		Paraspinous abscess
	Posterior elements	Osteomyelitis
Spinal canal	Epidural space	Epidural abscess
	Meninges	Meningitis
	Subdural space	Subdural abscess
	Spinal cord	Intramedullary abscess

Table 2.6-1
Anatomical description of spinal infections.

5   CAUSATIVE ORGANISMS

The spine can be infected by a vast array of organisms. Most commonly, it is due to pyogenic bacteria, of which *Staphylococcus aureus* accounts for more than 50% of the cases in reported series [5]. Mycobacterium tuberculosis is the most common nonpyogenic cause. Whilst being an uncommon cause of spinal infection in the UK, its incidence is increasing. **Table 2.6-2** lists the common agents.

However, a recent retrospective study by Collins et al [6] found that following instrumented spine surgery, the most frequently identified bacteria was *Propionibacterium*. **Table 2.6-3** summarizes their findings.

Gram-positive aerobic cocci	Staphylococcus aureus
	Staphylococcus (coagulase-negative)
	Streptococcus pyogenes
	Other streptococci
	Enterococci
Gram-negative aerobic cocci	Escherichia coli
	Proteus spp.
	Pseudomonas aeruginosa
	Klebsiella pneumoniae
	Salmonella spp.
Anaerobic bacteria	Propionibacterium spp.
	Bacteriodes fragilis
	Peptostreptococcus spp.
Other bacteria	Mycobacterium tuberculosis
	Brucella spp.
	Actinomyces israelii
Fungi	Aspergillus spp.
	Blastomyces dermatidiis
	Candida spp.
	Cryptococcus neoformans

Table 2.6-2
Agents causing spinal infections.

Bacteria	Frequency
Propionibacteria	34/80
Coagulase negative staphylococcus	19/80
Staphylococcus aureus	10/80
Methicillin-resistant staphylococcus aureus	8/80
Coliforms	3/80
Proteus	2/80
Diptheroids	2/80
Anaerobic streptococci	1/80
Alpha hemolytic streptococci	1/80

Table 2.6-3
Postoperative infections of the instrumented spine.

6   RISK FACTORS FOR SPINAL INFECTION

Clinicians should seek detailed histories from patients with suspected spinal infections as there are wide geographical variations in causative organisms. Furthermore, disease processes and drugs, be they prescription or recreational, can lead to infection with atypical organisms that will require special investigations to identify. Certain organisms such as propionibacteria and tuberculosis are difficult to culture and may take up to eight weeks.

Factors associated with spinal infection can be endogenous (patient related) such as age, immune status, smoking, and obesity, or exogenous, such as emergency surgery, and the type and duration of operation.

Of particular interest are the risk factors for patients undergoing spine surgery, many of which may lead to devastating complications. A review by Olsen et al [7] categorized the risks into preoperative, perioperative, and postoperative. **Table 2.6-4** identifies the main factors.

Preoperative	Perioperative	Postoperative
Age	Skin antisepsis	High blood sugars > 200 mg/dl
Body mass index (BMI)	Shaving	Postoperative CSF leak
Smoking	Type of operation	Incontinence
Nutritional status	Emergency operation	Transfusions (number and type)
Diabetes	Duration of operation	ITU stay
Malignancy	Durotomy	
Immunosuppressive drugs	Intraoperative hypothermia	
Transfusion (number and type)	Use of microscope, x-ray	
Previous spine surgery	Transfusion (number and type)	
Spinal cord compression	Other concurrent operations	
Incontinence		
Paralysis		
Recent injury/trauma		
Preoperative hospital stay		
ASA grade		

Table 2.6-4
Risk factors for surgical site infection.

On performing statistical analysis between the variables and an association with increased risk, their main conclusions were that obesity, postoperative incontinence, posterior approach, and tumor resections carried the greatest risk for surgical site infection.

7   DIAGNOSIS

The most frequent presenting complaint of spinal infection is pain. The pain is often related to movement or position, and varies greatly in intensity.

Constitutional symptoms are:

- fever,
- night sweats,
- anorexia,
- fatigue,
- weight loss (not usually present) [8].

Deformity tends to be a late-presenting feature, as there needs to be destabilization and destruction of the spinal elements for this to occur. Neurological deterioration is a rare presenting feature, but if apparent often represents epidural infection.

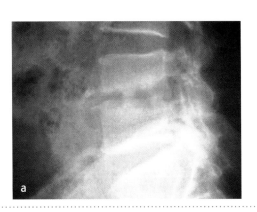
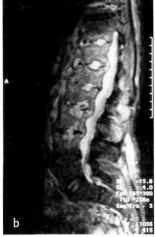

Fig 2.6-1a–b
a Lateral x-ray of a 64-year-old male with discitis.
b Lateral MRI of a patient with multilevel discitis.

Unfortunately, there are no diagnostic tests that are 100% reliable. Therefore, the diagnostic process must begin with a thorough history and clinical examination, so that investigations can be planned that will lead to the correct diagnosis. The history can be suggestive of the type of organism causing the infection, and thus is essential in helping guide the microbiologists.

Baseline investigations involve blood tests, looking for raised inflammatory markers such as erythrocyte sedimentation rate (ESR) and C-reactive protein (CRP), along with a full blood cell count. The ESR tends to be high in chronic bacterial infections, with the CRP being raised in both acute and chronic infections. The CRP, in addition, returns to normal quickly upon resolution of the infection, hence is a good marker of performance. The white blood cell (WBC) count is raised in under 40% of cases. Blood cultures need to be taken. Unfortunately, they are rarely positive.

Radiological assessment begins with plain x-rays. The features seen include disc space narrowing, irregularity of the vertebral end plates, defects in the subchondral bone and sclerosis. More rarely, paravertebral soft-tissue swellings can be seen. Such changes can take weeks to become apparent, hence, normal x-rays do not necessarily rule out spinal infection. Late features on plain x-ray include vertebral collapse, deformity, and bony fusion [5] (**Fig 2.6-1a**).

The next investigation of choice is magnetic resonance imaging (MRI) (**Fig 2.6-1b**). If this is unavailable, then computed tomography (CT) and myelography can be employed. MRI scans are the gold standard investigation. They have been shown to have a sensitivity of 96%, specificity of 92% and an accuracy of 94%. The sensitivity of an investigation indicates how successful it is in identifying patients suffering with a condition, in this case, spinal infection, as a percentage of all patients with the condition. In other words, MRI is accurate 96 times out of 100. A high sensitivity is desirable for a screening test. The specificity of an investigation indicates the success of identifying patients without the condition. A high specificity is desirable for a confirmatory test. Hence, MRI for spinal infections is a good screening and confirmatory test, hence, its high accuracy.

If doubt still remains as to the diagnosis, then radionucleotide scanning (bone scan) can be employed. Agents such as technetium-99m (^{99m}Tc) and indium-111-labelled white blood cells (^{111}In WBC) can be utilized.

Once the diagnosis of a spinal infection has been made, the hunt for the infective organism begins. If the blood cultures are negative and there is no pus discharging through the skin, then a biopsy of the infected tissue is required. This can be performed as a percutaneous or open technique. Helm et al [9] found that the use of a Harlow Wood bone biopsy trephine gave a diagnosis rate of 89% in suspected infections and 88% when the diagnosis was uncertain.

Isolation of the organism is a very important step in the management, as it guides the drug therapies. Special emphasis should be placed on the history taken from the patient. Certain bacteria, such as propionibacteria and mycobacteria require special microbiological tests, over extended periods of time, hence can be overlooked if an incomplete picture of the patient is provided.

8   TREATMENT

Treatments should be aimed at eradication of the infection, preserving neurological function and maintaining the mechanical integrity of the spinal column. This involves a combined effort by the spine surgeons, the microbiologists, and the radiologists. Prior to commencement of antibiotics, every effort must be taken to isolate the causative organism. If patients are very unwell, then empirical antibiotic therapy can be commenced, aimed at the most likely infectious agents.

Disc space infections can predominantly be treated with antibiotics. The clinical signs, the inflammatory markers, and microbiologists must guide the particular agent and the duration of treatment. In some instances, debridement and washout of the disc spaces can be performed. Patients may suffer from back pain, which can settle if the adjacent vertebrae fuse secondarily to the infection.

Vertebral osteomyelitis can also be treated initially with antibiotics. Indications for surgery include deformity and neurological compromise. The tuberculous spine, historically, has seen some heroic operations, such as the Hong Kong procedure (radical anterior debridement and autogenous strut grafting) [10]. However, antituberculous chemotherapy can be employed in the absence of deformity and neurological compromise (**Fig 2.6-2a–c**).

Abscesses around the spinal canal, such as epidural or subdural, usually employ surgical drainage as the mainstay of treatment, followed by antibiotics. However, patients who are systemically well with no neurological compromise, or those too sick to undergo surgery, can be treated with antibiotics alone.

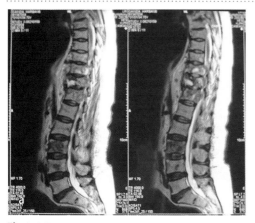
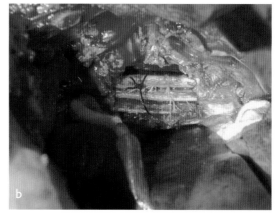
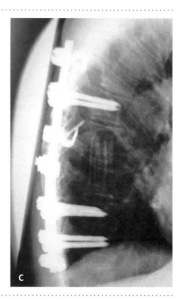

Fig 2.6-2a–c
a MRI of a 56-year-old male with tuberculosis.
b Strut graft in situ following anterior debridement.
c Postoperative x-ray.

8.1   ANTIBIOTIC PROPHYLAXIS IN SPINE SURGERY

Prevention is always preferable to the quest for a cure. Hence, all possible steps to avoid postoperative infections are taken (see chapter 3.1 Infection control and preventative precautions in the operating room). Such infections, although uncommon, can be catastrophic. Therefore, prophylactic antibiotics are used routinely. Evidence to support their use is not robust, although a recent metaanalysis concluded that their use is beneficial.

To keep postoperative infection risk to a minimum, prophylactic antibiotics should be employed, along with regular wound irrigation, intraoperatively using saline (with or without iodine). The use of drains should be kept to a minimum.

9   BIBLIOGRAPHY

1. **Calderone RR, Larsen JM** (1996) Overview and classifications of spinal infections. *Orthop Clin North Am;* 27(1):1–8.
2. **Breschet G** (1819) Easai sur les veines du rachis. Paris, Mequignon-Marvis.
3. **Rodet A** (1884) Experimental study on infectious osteomyelitis. *Compendium Readings of Academy of Science (France);* 569–571.
4. **Ozuna RM, Delamarter RB** (1996) Pyogenic vertebral osteomyelitis and postsurgical disc space infections. *Orthop Clin North Am;* 27(1):87–94.
5. **Sapico FL** (1996) Microbiology and antimicrobial therapy of spinal infections. *Orthop Clin North Am;* 27(1):9–13:
6. **Collins I, Burgoyne W, Chami G,** et al (2004) The management of infection following instrumented spinal surgery. Podium presentation, *Britspine;* Nottingham, UK
7. **Olsen MA, Mayfield J, Lauryssen C,** et al (2003) Risk factors for surgical site infection in spinal surgery. *J Neurosurg;* 98:149–155.
8. **Weinberg J, Silber JS** (2004) Infections of the spine: what the orthopedist needs to know. *Am J Orthop;* 33(1):13–17.
9. **Helm AT, Sell PJ, Lam KS** (2004) Accuracy of percutaneous Harlow Wood biopsies of vertebral lesions. Podium presentation, *Britspine;* Nottingham, UK.

2.7   PRECISION INJECTION TECHNIQUES FOR THE DIAGNOSIS AND TREATMENT OF SPINAL DISORDERS

1   INTRODUCTION

The history and physical examination of the spinal patient is of paramount importance in establishing a diagnosis. In the lumbar spine, one needs to establish whether the patient is complaining of pure axial low back pain or whether they have radicular pain due to mechanical compression and/or chemical irritation of a nerve root.

This sounds straightforward, however, in practice patients often present with both low back pain and leg pain. The leg pain may be referred from a degenerate disc or arthritic facet joint, or it may be radicular (originating from the nerve root).

Referred pain into the leg rarely goes beyond the knee and is primarily felt in the posterior thigh. Radicular pain, however, often goes beyond the knee into the calf and sole of the foot and may be associated with:

- numbness,
- pins and needles,
- tingling,
- weakness.

The physical examination may reveal a restriction in the straight leg raise for patients with radicular pain but not for those with referred pain.

Patients with low back pain maybe subdivided into those that have pain primarily arising from the disc, ie, discogenic pain, and those that have pain predominantly arising from the facet joint. Patients with discogenic pain will have pain on bending forward and increased discomfort when sitting. Patients with facet joint arthropathy will have pain that is aggravated by extension. A patient with advanced disc degeneration with significant loss of disc height may have a combination of both discogenic and facet joint pain. Young patients with tenderness in the L5/S1 region and pain on extension, particularly if they are keen sportspeople, may have a condition called spondylolysis which results from repeated stress injury to the pars interarticularis.

Kuslich et al reported on the tissue origin of low back pain [1]. In 193 consecutive patients undergoing decompressive surgery for herniated disc or spinal stenosis, by use of progressive local anesthesia and detailed observations, he was able to identify the site of back pain. In two third of patients the outer annulus of the intervertebral disc produced back pain that was similar to the low back pain suffered preoperatively. Stimulation of the facet capsule occasionally caused back pain, and stimulation of the swollen or compressed nerve root produced buttock or leg pain.

Patients of advanced years who have associated weight loss, night pain, a history of smoking, or cancer may have serious underlying pathology such as tumor, infection, or fracture.

Patients may be investigated with:

- plain x-rays,
- computed tomography (CT),
- isotope bone scans,
- single positron emission computed tomography (SPECT),
- magnetic resonance imaging (MRI) (**Fig 2.7-1a–b**).

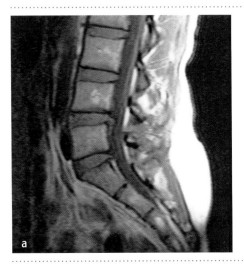 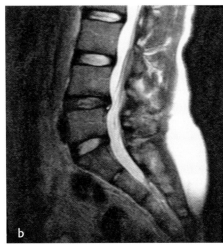

Fig 2.7-1a–b
a T1-weighted sagittal MRI scan of lumbar spine.
b T2-weighted sagittal MRI scan of lumbar spine. Note loss of hydration in L4/5 disc with high intensity zone posteriorly.

2   BIOPSY OF SPINAL TISSUE

MRI is the single most sensitive and most specific investigation for revealing disc herniation, soft-tissue or neurological lesions, tumor or infection. In the assessment of degenerative low back conditions, it has been shown to be too nonspecific to differentiate between patients with chronic low back pain and those without chronic low back pain [2].

Studies in asymptomatic individuals have shown "abnormal" MRI scans in up to 30–40% of cases [3, 4]. Even amongst symptomatic subjects, MRI findings of mild to moderate neural compromise, disc degeneration, disc bulge, and central canal stenosis were found not to correlate with the severity of symptoms [5]. It is often necessary to use precision injection techniques to assist in the diagnosis and treatment of such spinal disorders.

It is often necessary to perform a biopsy of spinal tissue, in particular where the diagnosis of infection and/or tumor is suspected from the MRI. Biopsies may be performed with the aid of CT scan, but difficulties within the CT scanner make the simultaneous administration of a general anesthetic difficult. As a result, biopsies in the CT scanner tend to be performed under local anesthetic using a Jamshedi needle. This technique is adequate for the biopsy of soft tissue; however, it is difficult to obtain core samples of bone. If these are required the radiologist may request that the spine surgeon carries out the biopsy under general anesthesia.

The spine surgeon often performs a biopsy using the Harlow Wood bone biopsy trephine. The larger size of this trephine necessitates that the patient has the procedure under a general anesthetic. The procedure is performed with the aid of fluoroscopy both in the AP and lateral plane on a radiolucent table. It is possible to safely biopsy the vertebral body and/or the disc using a percutaneous and posterolateral approach to the spine between T10 and the sacrum. If a biopsy is required above T10 it is safer to perform a direct posterior approach through the pedicle to avoid the risk of pneumothorax. These procedures may be carried out as a mini open procedure rather than a percutaneous procedure, as there is a risk to the spinal cord in such an approach. The alternative is to perform the biopsy under CT guidance.

In all cases, three separate cores of bone or disc material should be taken. Samples are sent to the microbiology department for microscopy, culture, and sensitivity plus culture for tuberculosis, and also sent to the pathology department for histology. A case of tumor in the spine has been described with coincident infection. Therefore, it is of paramount importance to send specimens for histopathology and microbiological assessment. The accuracy of percutaneous Harlow Wood biopsy has been reported as achieving a diagnosis in 88% of cases with a sensitivity of 87% and a specificity of 100% [6].

3   INJECTIONS FOR LOW BACK PAIN

3.1   FACET JOINT INJECTIONS

The lumbar facet joints are a potential source of low back pain and referred leg pain. The term facet syndrome is characterized by pain and tenderness in the region of the lower lumbar facet joints; pain is aggravated by extension and may be referred to the posterior thigh but rarely goes beyond the knee.

The prevalence of facet joint involvement in low back pain varies between 15–40%, with back pain caused solely by the facets in only 7%. It must be accepted that a degree of disc degeneration will always be present with facet joint degeneration. However the relative contributions to low back pain by either the facet joint or the intervertebral disc vary allowing triage of patients into predominate facet joint pain or predominate discogenic pain.

Facet joint pain may be treated with facet blocks. These are performed with the patient awake and under local anesthesia. The patient is placed in the prone position. The C-arm may be used to check that adequate AP and lateral views can be obtained. The skin is prepped and draped, then a local anesthetic (1% lignocaine hydrochloride) is infiltrated in the skin and a 0.9 × 125 mm spinal needle is inserted, targeting the L4/5 and L5/S1 facet joints in the AP projection. Once the needle hits bone the C-arm is swung into an oblique projection which will show the facet joints more clearly. Final adjustments of the needle tip are made. Some surgeons prefer to inject a contrast agent to verify needle tip position; others simply accept the position on the biplane fluoroscopy. A mixture of 10 ml of 0.25% bupivacaine and 80 mg of triamcinolone is divided into four (ie, 2.5 ml for each joint) and injected into each of the lower four facet joints. If the clinical situation dictates, the L3/4 facet joints may also be injected. The patient can experience 3–4 months of significant pain relief and in some instances this may extend to six months. The injection is likely to be both diagnostic and therapeutic but not curative.

3.2   MEDIAL BRANCH BLOCKS

The facet joints are innervated by the medial branch of the posterior primary ramus. The anterior primary ramus is the main nerve trunk that supplies various myotomes and dermatomes in the leg. By using different needle placement it is possible to selectively block the medial branch of the posterior primary ramus. This temporarily blocks the innervation of the facet joints concerned and serves as a useful diagnostic test.

A standard 0.9 × 125 mm spinal needle may be used, but due to overlap in innervation the lower three facet joints need to be blocked (ie, L3/4, L4/5, and L5/S1) on each side. The needle tip is placed precisely at the junction of the transverse process and the superior articular facet of L4 and L5. At the sacrum the needle tip is placed over the ala of the sacrum in close contact to the articular facet medially. It is necessary to take a lateral x-ray to confirm that the needle has not been placed too deeply, in which case the needle would be in close proximity

to the neural foramen where the anterior primary ramus exits. If this is the case the needle should be withdrawn to the correct place. 1 ml of 1% lignocaine hydrochloride with 1 ml of 0.25% bupivacaine is injected at each of the six sites. The patient is asked to keep a pain diary over the following few days. If the procedure is successful in temporarily relieving the back pain, then a facet joint denervation may be performed to produce more lasting pain relief.

3.3   FACET JOINT DENERVATION

This technique aims to denervate the facet joints of the lower lumbar spine by destroying the medial branch of the posterior primary ramus at L3/4, L4/5, and L5/S1 bilaterally. When considering radio frequency denervation it is logical that a medial branch block is a more appropriate diagnostic tool than a simple facet joint block because it directly evaluates the structure scheduled for ablation [8].

Under aseptic conditions, with the patient in the prone position on a radiolucent table, the levels to be denervated are located by AP fluoroscopy. The target point (ie, the base of the transverse process where it meets the root of the superior articular process) is marked on the skin. The L5 posterior ramus courses in the grove between ala and the superior articular facet of S1 and is approached with the probe lying parallel to the posterior primary ramus proper as it hooks over the sacrum.

The skin is anesthetized with 1% lignocaine hydrochloride and three Sluijter Mehta Kit (SMK) needles are inserted to their appropriate target point on one side. When AP and lateral fluoroscopy show the needle tips to be appropriately positioned the needle is connected via a sterile lead to the radio frequency generator (**Fig 2.7-2a–b**).

Following this, a period of sensory and motor stimulation will be undergone to check final needle position. The patient must be fully awake and able to cooperate during this part of the procedure. Sensory stimulation is performed at 100 Hz up to 1 V. The patient may experience typical low back pain during this; indeed some surgeons actually record the voltage threshold when the patient experiences low back pain. Motor stimulation then follows. The radio frequency generator is set at 2 Hz and the voltage is slowly increased to 2 V. If motor stimulation of the corresponding myotomes occurs (ie, the foot is seen to twitch) then the needle must be repositioned.

When the SMK needle is correctly positioned it is usual to see contraction of the ipsilateral multifidus during motor stimulation. Provided satisfactory sensory and motor stimulation has occurred (the patient has not experienced radicular pain and there is no evidence of muscle activity in the foot or ankle) then the surgeon may proceed with performing the lesion. Most surgeons will lesion at 80°C for 2 minutes at each level. Once all three levels have been completed on the right hand side the procedure is repeated on the left.

Van Kleef et al performed a randomized trial of radio frequency lumbar facet denervation for chronic low back pain in 31 patients [9]. All patients had a positive response to a diagnostic medial branch block and were subsequently randomized to one of two treatment groups. Patients in the radio frequency treatment group (n=15) received an 80°C radio frequency lesion of the posterior ramus of the segmental nerve roots L3, L4, and L5. Patients in the control group (n=16) underwent the same procedure but without use of the radio frequency current. Both the treating physician and the patient were blinded to the group assignment.

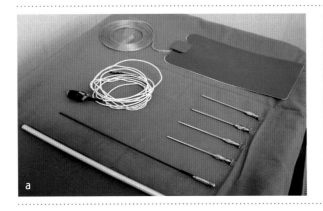
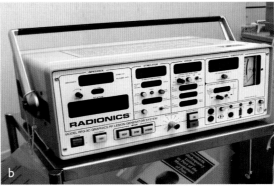

Fig 2.7-2a–b
a Equipment required for facet rhizolysis.
b Radio frequency generator.

The authors concluded that radio frequency lumbar zygapoph-yseal joint denervation resulted in a significant alleviation of pain and functional disability in a selected group of patients with chronic low back pain, both on a short-term and a long-term basis. It is thought that radio frequency denervation may provide relief of facet joint pain for up to two years.

3.4   PARS BLOCK IN SPONDYLOLYSIS

The reported incidence of symptomatic defects of the pars in the general population is approximately 5%. This is consid-erably higher in young athletes, varying from 15–47%.

The diagnosis may have been made on:

- plain x-rays,
- SPECT scan,
- reverse-gantry CT scan, or
- MRI scan.

However, the stress fracture of the pars articulares may be old and in order to ascertain whether this is the cause of symp-toms, it is sometimes useful to perform a pars block under fluoroscopic control.

Under aseptic conditions a 0.9 × 125 mm spinal needle is placed in the region of the pars parallel to the orientation of the L5/S1 disc. Once satisfactory placement of the needle has been con-firmed, 1 ml of radiopaque contrast agent is injected to verify needle position. The contrast agent may outline the capsule of the facet joint as the pars defect often communicates with the facet joint. 1 ml of 0.25% bupivacaine with 40 mg of triam-cinolone is then injected into each defect assuming a bilateral pars defect.

The patient is interviewed two weeks after receiving the injec-tion and asked if the injection has provided symptomatic relief. If so, the patient may be offered surgery to repair such a defect assuming there is no concomitant disc degeneration on the MRI scan.

3.5   PROVOCATIVE LUMBAR DISCOGRAPHY

MRI scan of the lumbosacral spine often reveals abnormalities within the disc. The commonest appearance is loss of hydra-tion indicating early degeneration of the disc.

There may be a high intensity zone situated posteriorly in the disc. This shows up as a bright signal on the T2-weighted scan (see 1 Introduction, **Fig 2.7-1b**, in this chapter) and is thought to represent a tear in the posterior annulus. Modic changes in the lumbar end plate and surrounding subchondral bone have been described in detail, but similarly their significance re-mains unclear. None of the above findings necessarily indicate that this disc is symptomatic and responsible for the patient's low back pain.

The purpose of lumbar discography is to determine whether the intervertebral disc is indeed the source of pain. The basic premise of this investigation is that placing a needle in a nor-mal disc and filling that disc with fluid will not produce pain. The technique remains controversial, with many authors re-porting both false positive and false negative results. Other authors stress the influence of psychosocial factors on pain perception.

The procedure is carried out under a light neuroleptic anes-thetic (conscious sedation). The patient is placed prone on a radiolucent table. If lordosis is extreme it may help to place a pillow under the lower abdomen and pelvis to reverse this. The patient is prepared and draped.

The abnormal discs on MRI scan are targeted, and it is important to pick an adjacent disc that appears normal on MRI scan chosen to serve as a control. At L5/S1 with the C-arm in the AP plane, the gantry is tilted so that it is exactly parallel with the end plates of L5 and S1. Once achieved, the image intensifier is then moved into an oblique projection. This projection should reveal a safe porthole into the L5/S1 disc through a triangle bordered by the iliac crest laterally, the superior articular process medially and the inferior end plate of L5 superiorly.

Using a 0.9 × 125 mm spinal needle and a standard posterolateral approach the centre of this triangle is targeted, allowing the needle to pass in line with the x-ray beam. Once the needle approaches the disc a smaller 0.45 mm × 150 mm spinal needle

is prepared by placing a gentle curve at the tip using a syringe and piece of gauze in line with the bevel of the needle. This will allow more midline placement of the needle tip. The 0.45 mm needle is inserted through the 0.9 mm needle, with its curve facing medially. Care should be taken not to touch the tip of this needle. The needle is advanced and ideally positioned in the centre of the nucleus. This two-needle technique has been shown to reduce the risk of infection. Inaccurate placement in the annulus may provide a false positive discogram result and should be avoided.

Antibiotic prophylaxis should consist of 900 mg intravenous cephradine and 100 mg intradiscal cephradine. 100 mg of cephradine is inserted into the contrast agent prior to injection of the disc. In this way, a high concentration of antibiotic enters the disc, reducing the risk of infection still further.

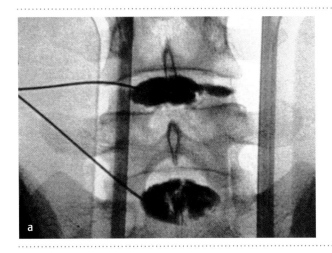
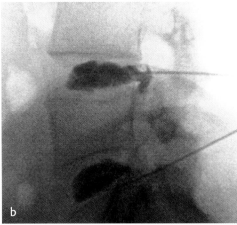

Fig 2.7-3a–b
a AP x-rays postdiscography at L4/5 and L5/S1.
b Lateral x-ray postdiscography at the same levels.
Note spread of contrast into the posterior annulus at L4/5 (Adams morphology grade IV).

If it is not possible to enter the L5/S1 disc, the surgeon may try a posterolateral approach from the opposite side. In a similar fashion, the remaining target discs, for example L3/4 and L4/5, are cannulated. In addition a control disc (one that appears to be normal on the MRI scan) is cannulated (**Fig 2.7-3a–b**). Once all the required discs are cannulated the anesthetist is instructed to lighten the sedation.

Each disc is then prefilled with up to 1 ml of contrast agent (containing antibiotic). The disc that is thought to be asymptomatic is tested first by applying firm and gentle pressure on the syringe. The patient is asked to grade the pain on a scale of 0 to 5. This scale does not represent the severity of pain, rather, it represents the quality of pain. The number 5 represents an exact replica of the patient's usual chronic low back pain. The number 0 represents the exact opposite, ie, a totally new pain experience for the patient. AP and lateral fluoroscopy is carried out to show the pattern of contrast within the disc. The process is repeated for all discs concerned and the results are tabulated recording the morphology of the disc according to Adam [10].

This classification describes:

- Grade I as cotton-ball appearance
- Grade II as lobular
- Grade III as irregular
- Grade IV as fissured
- Grade V as ruptured

Grade I and II are considered normal, while III to V are considered abnormal. The volume of contrast agent injected, the pressure (low, medium, or high), and the pain concordance (0 to 5) should be recorded. If uncertainty exists it may be necessary to interrogate each disc again. By the end of the procedure

it is usually possible to have a good idea if the target disc is responsible for the patient's pain.

Simple discography has been shown to improve surgical outcome. However, Madan et al found that after circumferential fusion clinical outcome rates with and without discography were not statistically different [11]. Derby et al, with the aid of pressure control discography, described a "chemically sensitive disc" that provoked pain at very low pressure and a "mechanically sensitive disc" that reproduced pain at higher pressures [12]. Patients subsequently went on to either anterior interbody fusion or intertransverse fusion. Those patients with chemically sensitive discs did well following anterior interbody fusion. However, those patients with chemically sensitive discs who underwent intertransverse fusion did poorly. He concluded that those patients with chemically sensitive discs should have a disc ablative procedure.

It is disappointing that MRI findings such as the high intensity zone or modic changes in the adjacent end plate are unable to predict the results of surgical outcome. As such, the role of provocative lumbar discography remains vitally important in selecting patients appropriate for spinal fusion and total disc replacement.

3.6   INTRADISCAL ELECTROTHERMAL THERAPY (IDET)

IDET was introduced as a treatment for those patients who failed conservative care, including physical therapy, and who otherwise would have proceeded to spinal fusion.

The procedure involves a light neuroleptic anesthetic and the passage of a catheter into a discographically proven symptomatic disc. The catheter has a 5 cm terminal section that is not insulated and when connected to a generator will allow a controlled amount of thermal energy to be released to the disc.

The catheter is navigated into the ideal position using the AP and lateral fluoroscopy (**Fig 2.7-4a–b**); an additional view (Ferguson view) is used (maximal caudal tilt of x-ray beam) to verify appropriate catheter deployment. A standard heating protocol is used with the catheter slowly brought up to the final temperature of 90°C and held at this temperature for four minutes. Total treatment time for each disc is 16.5 minutes. The catheter is carefully removed and 100 mg of cephradine is injected into the disc before removal of the introduced needle. The patient is recovered and allowed home the same day but must wear a lumbosacral orthosis for a period of 6 weeks.

Targeted thermal energy has been shown to:

• shrink collagen fibrils,
• cauterize granulation tissue,
• coagulate nerve tissue.

IDET may coagulate annular nociceptors and lead to contraction of collagen.

Freeman et al have shown adequate temperatures in an in vivo animal to theoretically perform both coagulation of nociceptors and contraction of collagen [13]. However, this group subsequently was not able to show denervation of an experimentally-induced posterior annular lesion in sheep following IDET [14]. It would appear the exact mechanism of action has yet to be explained.

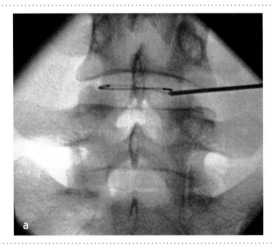
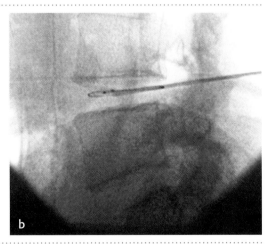

Fig 2.7-4a–b
a AP x-ray.
b Lateral x-ray.
Both x-rays show final IDET
catheter position at L4/5.

There are two randomized controlled studies reporting on the efficacy of IDET:

- Pauza et al [15] conclude IDET to be an effective treatment for discogenic low back pain with modest improvement in outcome scores.
- Freeman et al [16] in a randomized double-blind controlled clinical trial, showed no significant benefit from IDET over placebo.

It is clear from the literature that the procedure is of marginal benefit for a highly selected group of patients, and is not beneficial for the vast majority of patients with chronic discogenic low back pain.

3.7   MANIPULATION OF THE COCCYX AND SACROCOCCYGEAL INJECTION

Patients with nontraumatic sacrococcygeal pain should be offered simple analgesics and the use of a pressure-relieving cushion initially. If symptoms persist patients may be offered a manipulation of the coccyx and injection of the sacrococcygeal joint under general anesthetic.

The procedure is done with the patient in the left lateral position. The skin is prepared and draped. The surgeon prepares an injection of 5 ml of 0.25% bupivacaine with 40 mg of triamcinolone. A rectal examination is performed with the coccyx being grasped between the index finger and thumb of the right hand. The orientation of the coccyx is noted and the coccyx manipulated through a full range of motion at the sacrococcygeal joint. The surgeon then uses his left hand to inject the solution to the sacrococcygeal joint and not beyond. Great care is taken not to advance the needle into the rectum, as clearly contamination and infection could occur. If the patient benefits from the injection but the symptoms recur they may be offered a second injection. If symptoms return following this, consideration could be given to a coccygectomy.

3.8   SACROILIAC JOINT INJECTIONS

The sacroiliac joint may be a cause of chronic low back pain. The patient typically describes unilateral pain when standing on the affected side. Sacroiliac joint syndrome may follow an L4 to S1 spinal fusion as there is extra stress applied to the sacroiliac joint. The syndrome may be recognized by a positive forced abduction and external rotation (FABER) test. Plain radiographs may show unilateral sclerosis of the sacroiliac joint.

The patient is placed in the prone position, the left hip is raised approximately 10–30° from the table with a pillow for visualizing the right sacroiliac joint, or the right hip is raised similarly for visualizing the left sacroiliac joint. The patient's position is adjusted until the anterior and posterior orifices of the caudal one third of the joint are seen to be superimposed, which orientates the sides of the caudal one third of the joint parallel to the x-ray beam. The prone/oblique position of the patient uncovers the posterior orifice of the joint and allows direct entry into the joint using a vertically-oriented needle.

The sacral area is prepared and draped; the soft tissues are infiltrated with local anesthetic. Under fluoroscopic control a standard 0.9 × 125 mm spinal needle is then superimposed on the caudal one third of the joint midway between the sides of the joint. The needle is introduced into the soft tissues and directed perpendicular to the fluoroscopy table and parallel to the x-ray beam. The needle may meet resistance initially; this can be overcome as the needle enters the posterior sacroiliac ligament. On average the needle is inserted approximately 3–5 cm from the skin surface.

A lateral x-ray is taken to confirm the appropriate depth of the needle in the joint. 1 ml of radiopaque contrast is then injected into the joint. The contrast material should outline the margins of the joint. A mixture of 5 ml of 0.25% bupivacaine and 40 mg of triamcinolone is then injected into the joint space. The patient is interviewed after two weeks to assess the efficacy of the injection. If symptoms recur a repeat injection may be offered and in rare instances if the symptoms remain and are significantly disabling, the patient may be offered a sacroiliac fusion.

3.9   INTRAARTICULAR INJECTION OF THE HIP JOINT

It is not uncommon for patients with degenerative disc disease in the lumbar spine to have concomitant osteoarthritis in the hip. This can pose a diagnostic difficulty particularly when symptoms of low back pain overlap with pain radiating into the groin or hip. One useful technique is a diagnostic intraarticular injection of the hip joint. The patient's response to this injection will ascertain the primary source of pain: either L5 nerve root compromise in the spine or osteoarthritis in the hip.

The procedure is carried out under strict aseptic conditions with the patient supine. The skin is prepared and draped and with the aid of an image intensifier in AP projection, a needle is placed perpendicular to the x-ray beam with the tip of the needle in the centre of the femoral head (**Fig 2.7-5**).

The skin is infiltrated with 2 ml of 1% lignocaine hydrochloride. The surgeon then palpates the femoral artery and, avoiding this, inserts the needle in direct alignment with the x-ray beam toward the exact centre of the femoral head. When the needle contacts bone it is necessary to ascertain that the needle is intraarticular and 1–2 ml of radiopaque contrast is then injected. This should produce an arthrogram if the needle is properly placed. If the tip of the needle is not in the joint the contrast material will form a puddle at the tip and may be resting on the overlying acetabulum. Once intraarticular placement has been confirmed, 10 ml of 0.25% bupivacaine and 80 mg of triamcinolone is injected into the joint. The needle is removed; the femoral artery is palpated once again. The hip is then moved through flexion and internal/external rotation to allow the anesthetic and steroid to travel around in the joint.

The patient is interviewed at two weeks following the injection. If the hip and groin pain has resolved then consideration should be given to hip replacement before any spine surgery. If on the other hand the injection has not helped, careful

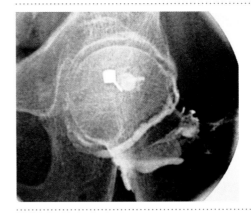

Fig 2.7-5
Intraarticular injection left hip. Note intracapsular spread of contrast.

attention to a spinal cause for the hip and groin pain should follow. If doubt exists it is often helpful in this situation to perform a L5 nerve root block.

3.10 INJECTION OF THE TROCHANTERIC BURSA

Trochanteric bursitis may be confused with low back pain, with radiation to the lateral aspect of the thigh. It is easily diagnosed by pinpoint tenderness over the trochanteric bursa. If doubt exists about the origin of the pain, a diagnostic injection of the trochanteric bursa can help elucidate the cause.

This injection must be carried out under strict aseptic conditions. The skin is prepared and draped and then using a needle and a syringe with 10 ml of 0.25% bupivacaine and 40 mg of triamcinolone the most tender point over the greater trochanter is injected with the bupivacaine/triamcinolone mixture.

4 INJECTIONS FOR SCIATICA

Radiculopathy may be due to a prolapsed intervertebral disc (**Fig 2.7-6a–b**) or lateral recess stenosis. Studies on the pathophysiology of sciatica suggest that mechanical deformation of the nerve roots is responsible at least in part for the symptom of pain. In addition, biological activity of disc tissue has been shown to injure nerve roots by exciting an intense inflammatory response further contributing to pain.

70% of patients with radiologically-proven disc prolapse report a decrease in pain and 60% return to work within four weeks of initial conservative management. Physical therapy in the form of McKenzie exercises may help but for those who have persistent symptoms an epidural injection of local anesthetic and steroid can reduce the inflammatory response leading to a reduction in pain thus obviating the need for surgery. Similarly, for those patients with spinal stenosis an epidural may be effective in reducing leg pain, although it is generally thought to be less effective when compared to patients with

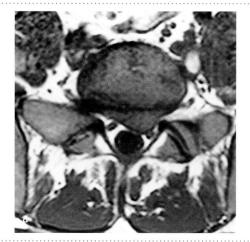 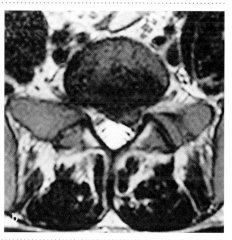

Fig 2.7-6a–b
a Axial T1 MRI.
b Axial T2 MRI.
Both axial MRI scans showing left-sided L5/S1 disc prolapse.

disc prolapse. Clearly if the patient has defined motor weakness in a specific myotome or signs or symptoms of cauda equina syndrome then an urgent surgical decompression should be considered.

4.1   CAUDAL EPIDURAL INJECTION

Caudal epidural injection may be performed without the need for imaging. However, in the obese patient it can be of value to have a lateral fluoroscopic picture to localize the sacral hiatus. The patient can be placed in either the left lateral position or the prone position. The sacral hiatus is palpated and marked with a permanent marker.

The skin is prepared and draped, and using a 0.9 × 125 mm spinal needle the sacral hiatus is approached. There will be a sudden loss of resistance. If imaging is used, a small amount of contrast is injected. A lateral x-ray will show the contrast outlining the epidural space. A high volume of fluid is required with 20 ml of 0.125% bupivacaine combined with 80 mg of triamcinolone.

The injection is given slowly and the patient's blood pressure monitored at 15-minute intervals for 1 hour. If the patient has symptoms limited to the left leg they should remain in the lateral position with the left leg down to maximize the travel of the medication to the affected side. It is unlikely that a caudal epidural will be as effective for an L3/4 disc prolapse as compared to an L5/S1 disc prolapse simply due to the distance the medication has to travel.

4.2   LUMBAR EPIDURAL INJECTION

Lumbar epidural injections are performed generally by the anesthetists as they have more experience with this route of administration. The patient may be placed in the lateral position or sitting up with the spine in as much flexion as possible. The spine is palpated and the L3/4 level marked. The skin is prepared and draped; using a standard epidural needle the epidural space is located by the loss-of-resistance method. A mixture of 10 ml of 0.125% bupivacaine and 40 mg of triamcinolone is injected into the epidural space. The patient is placed with the symptomatic leg in the lowermost position for recovery. Blood pressures are checked every 15 minutes for 1 hour.

4.3   TARGETED FORAMINAL EPIDURAL STEROID INJECTION

For patients with unilateral radicular symptoms who have undergone MRI and had a clear diagnosis made, the use of targeted foraminal epidural steroid injection should be considered to relieve leg pain. The procedure is carried out under local anesthetic, with the patient prone using a standard posterolateral approach to the relevant foramen. It is important to inject at the level of the disc pathology. For example, an L5/S1 disc prolapse will compromise the S1 nerve root. A targeted foraminal epidural steroid injection carried out at the level of the disc will outline the epidural space and cover both the L5 and the S1 nerve roots. An L5 nerve root block carried out high in the foramen will not necessarily treat the symptoms of an L5/S1 disc prolapse because the S1 nerve root may not be covered.

The patient is placed prone and the skin prepared and draped. To begin, the image intensifier is used in the AP position. Using a 0.9 × 125 mm spinal needle the respective foramen is targeted. Checks are made both on the AP and lateral x-rays. Care is taken not to inadvertently puncture the disc; if this does occur then intravenous antibiotics should be administered to reduce the risk of discitis. The needle should be very slowly advanced in the AP projection traveling below the pedicle. Ideally, the needle should be finally positioned just medial to the 6-o'clock position of the pedicle. Contrast should be seen to enhance the epidural space and the exiting nerve root (**Fig 2.7-7a–b**). Once a satisfactory needle tip position has been obtained, a mixture of 4 ml of 0.25% bupivacaine and 40 mg of triamcinolone should, be injected. Due to the low volume and accuracy of injection it is not usually necessary to monitor blood pressure.

The outcome of targeted foraminal epidural steroid injection for radicular pain has been studied [17]. In this series of 83 consecutive patients 74.7% of cases at a median of 20 months were able to avoid surgical intervention (decompression/discectomy).

4.4   CHEMONUCLEOLYSIS FOR LUMBAR DISC HERNIATION

Chemonucleolysis was the first injection used and made up from a purified extract of the papaya fruit; this was injected into the disc to treat intervertebral disc prolapse. Its reputation was damaged because of complications that generally turned out to be due to either poor technique of needle placement or to unrecognized comorbidity.

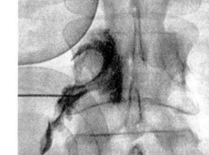 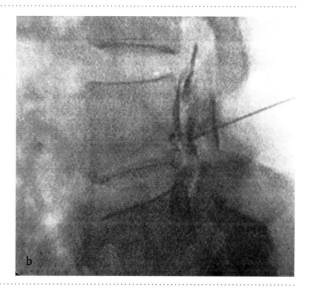

Fig 2.7-7a–b
a   AP x-ray.
b   Lateral x-ray shows final needle position after L4/5 foraminal epidural steroid injection. Contrast outlines the L4 nerve root and surrounding epidural space.

Intradural injection of the enzyme with serious neurological sequelae has occurred but experienced radiological technique should make this complication extremely unlikely. There was also anxiety in the United States because of the risk of anaphylaxis. The most serious complication of chemonucleolysis is transverse myelitis. This occurs in between 1 in 18,000 and 1 in 25,000 cases. There has been renewed interest in the technique, particularly in younger patients. The procedure is preceded by a lumbar discogram with AP and lateral x-rays to confirm precise needle placement with radiopaque contrast. Once precision needle placement has been obtained, the chymopapain is slowly injected and the needle removed. There is risk of anaphylaxis.

4.5   ELECTROTHERMAL DISC DECOMPRESSION

Electrothermal disc decompression is a new technique initially developed by Oratec, the company responsible for the release of IDET. The IDET catheter has been modified to achieve focal thermal treatment of a contained disc herniation (**Fig 2.7-8**).

The catheter is introduced into the region of the disc prolapse using fluoroscopy. Once in place the catheter is connected to a generator and heat is applied to the disc. It is proposed that this heat leads to a volume reduction at the site of the disc herniation thereby relieving neural compression and leg pain.

A cadaveric study looked at the acute biomechanical effects of such a catheter on cadaveric human lumbar discs [18]. The study showed that there was a 35% reduction in the magnitude of stress peaks in the posterior annulus following treatment with the catheter. Clinical studies have been limited. Deen et al reported a prospective study of ten patients with intractable radicular symptoms and unilateral contained lumbar disc protrusions that were treated with electrothermal disc decompression using such a catheter [19]. In this small series of patients, electrothermal disc decompression did not result in any meaningful decrease in the size of the disc protrusion, nor did it produce satisfactory relief of radicular symptoms. As such, this device remains unproven for the treatment of radicular symptoms.

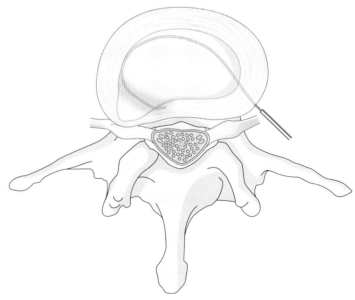

Fig 2.7-8

Axial cross section showing decompression catheter with terminal catheter located in the region of the disc prolapse.

4.6   OZONE CHEMONUCLEOLYSIS

The use of oxygen/ozone in medicine dates back to the WWI when it was used in an attempt to treat gangrene in wounds from firearms. Since 1995 it has been used to reduce the volume of disc prolapse and the associated compression of adjacent nerves. The use of medical ozone is not widespread and clearly further studies are required on the possible mechanism of action and the efficacy when compared to natural history and other available treatments.

4.7   ANTI-TNF-α THERAPY

Evidence from animal studies indicates that TNF-α plays a role in the pathophysiology of sciatica. In one pilot study, infliximab was administered intravenously. Promising results were achieved, with significant reduction in leg pain sustained at three months by patients.

5   INJECTIONS FOR AXIAL NECK PAIN

Neck pain may be conveniently divided into that predominantly arising from the disc (discogenic pain) or that arising predominantly from the facet joints (facet joint pain). Patients who complain predominantly of pain on flexion are more likely to have discogenic pain, and those that complain of pain on extension are more likely to have facet joint pain.

5.1   FACET JOINT INJECTION

Facet joint injections may be carried out under local anesthesia with the patient in the prone position and with the aid of the image intensifier. Local anesthesia is employed and a 0.9 × 125 mm spinal needle is used from a direct posterior approach. The needles are usually angled to follow the alignment of the facet joints in the cervical spine (45° craniocaudal tilt). The commonest sites of facet joint degeneration are at C5/6 and C6/7. Injections are usually carried out bilaterally with a mixture of 10 ml of 0.25% bupivacaine mixed with 40–80 mg of triamcinolone divided between four joints. The patient can expect a temporary relief of extension-related neck pain. During this pain-free period it is helpful to increase the range of motion through physiotherapy and restore cervical lordosis.

5.2   FACET JOINT DENERVATION

Patients demonstrating a good but short-lived response to facet joint injections may be offered a facet joint denervation performed with a radio frequency generator and standard SMK needles.

6   INJECTIONS FOR ARM PAIN OR BRACHALGIA

5.3   CERVICAL DISCOGRAPHY

Where doubt remains regarding the source of axial neck pain, cervical discography may be employed. It is more technically demanding in the cervical spine because an anteromedial approach is employed. The presence of the esophagus, trachea, and carotid sheath make precise needle placement somewhat hazardous.

The procedure may be carried out under local anesthesia, again employing a two-needle technique. Antibiotic prophylaxis should consist of both intravenous and intradiscal antibiotics. The pain provocation often results in bizarre patterns of radiation into the jaw and face etc.

Some authors describe cervical discography as unreliable. There appears to be less literature regarding the prediction of surgical outcome for patients undergoing fusion or disc replacement following cervical discography.

6.1   TARGETED FORAMINAL EPIDURAL STEROID INJECTION

Local corticosteroid injections may be indicated in patients who have persistent radicular pain. These may be delivered by the anterolateral approach or the direct lateral approach. The technique is performed under fluoroscopic guidance and strict asepsis. Patients may be positioned in an upright sitting position or the supine position. A lateral x-ray is performed. A typical case might involve a posterolateral disc protrusion at C5/6 with the patient complaining of a left C6 radiculopathy.

In this case the surgeon would line the spinal needle up against the anterosuperior margin of the C6 posterior articular process. The needle is advanced after infiltration of local anesthesia. Once the tip of the needle has reached the bone it is slowly displaced and advanced 5–10 mm anteriorly towards the intervertebral foramen. AP and oblique views help in final positioning.

After careful aspiration to exclude blood or cerebral spinal fluid, 40 mg of triamcinolone plus 3 ml of 0.125% bupivacaine mixture is slowly injected. It is wise to have some monitoring (pulse oximetry) in place when performing this procedure. Postoperatively, the patient's blood pressure and pulse must be carefully observed and recorded every 15 minutes for at least 1 hour.

6.2   SUBACROMIAL INJECTION

On occasion, patients presenting with neck and shoulder tip pain may have pathology within the shoulder joint. It is important to include the shoulder in the clinical examination. Patients who complain of a "painful arc" may have subacromial impingement. In these cases it is helpful to perform a diagnostic and therapeutic injection using 10 ml of 0.25% bupivacaine and 40 mg of triamcinolone in the subacromial region.

6.3   INJECTIONS FOR CARPAL TUNNEL SYNDROME

Patients who have referred pain into the thumb, index, and middle finger should be suspected of having this syndrome. This condition may coexist with radiculopathy due to C5/6 or C6/7 disc prolapse. In this situation the patient's symptoms are exacerbated by the double-crush syndrome. Nerve conduction studies may assist in the diagnosis. These may reveal marked slowing of the conduction velocity in the median nerve across the wrist confirming the diagnosis. If carpal tunnel syndrome is coexistent with cervical radiculopathy, the median nerve compression should be dealt with first. A trial injection of local anesthesia and steroid into the carpal tunnel under the flexor retinaculum may be both diagnostic and therapeutic. If symptoms recur the patient should be considered for carpal tunnel decompression.

7   BIBLIOGRAPHY

1. **Kuslich SD, Ulstrom CL, Michael CJ** (1991) The tissue origin of low back pain and sciatica: A report of pain response to tissue stimulation during operations on the lumbar spine using local anesthesia. *Orthop Clin N Am;* 22(2): 181–187.

2. **Carragee EJ, Hannibal M** (2004) Diagnostic evaluation of low back pain. *Orthop Clin N Am;* 35(1): 7–16.

3. **Boden S, Davis D, Dina T, et al** (1990) Abnormal magnetic resonance scans of the lumbar spine in asymptomatic subjects. A prospective investigation. *J Bone Joint Surg;* 72(8): 403–408.

4. **Jensen M, Brant-Zawadzki M, Obuchowski N,** et al (1994) Magnetic *Eng J Med;* 331(2): 69–73.

5. **Beattie PF, Meyers S,P Stratford P, et al** (2000) Associations between patient report of symptoms and anatomic impairment visible on lumbar MR imaging. *Spine;* 25(7): 819–828.

6. **Helm AT, Sell PJ, Lam KS** (2005) Accuracy of percutaneous Harlow Wood biopsies of vertebral lesions. *J Bone J Surg (Br);* Orth Proceedings Suppl III; 87-B:240.

7. **Schwarzer AC, Wang S, Bogduk N, et al** (1995) Prevalence and clinical features of lumbar zygapophysial joint pain: A study in an Australian population with chronic low back pain. *Am Rheum Dis;* 54(2): 100–106.

8. **Hall DJ** (2004) Facet joint denervation: A minimally invasive treatment for low back pain in selected patients. *Herkowitz HN (ed). The Lumbar Spine,* Official Publication of the ISSLS, 3rd ed. Philadelphia: Lippincott Williams & Wilkins, 307–311.

9. **Van Kleef M, Barendse G, Kessels A, et al** (1999) Randomised trial of radio frequency lumbar facet denervation for chronic low back pain. *Spine;* 24(18): 1937–1942.

10. **Agorastides ID, Lam KS, Freeman BJ, et al** (2002) The Adams classification for cadaveric discograms: inter– and intraobserver error in the clinical setting. *European Spine Journal;* 11(1): 76–79.

11. **Madan S, Gundanna M, Harley JM, et al** (2002) Does provocative discography screening of discogenic low back pain improve surgical outcome? *J Spinal Disord Tech;* 15(3): 245–251.

12. **Derby R, Howard M, Grant J, et al** (1999) The ability of pressure controlled discography to predict surgical and nonsurgical outcome. *Spine;* 24: 364–371.

13. **Freeman BJC, Walters R, Moore RJ, et al** (2001) In-vivo measurement of peak posterior annular and nuclear temperatures obtained during Intradiscal Electrothermal Therapy (IDET) in sheep. *Podium presentation at 28th Annual meeting of ISSLS,* Edinburgh, Scotland.

14. **Freeman BJC, Walters RM, Moore RJ, et al** (2003) Does intradiscal electrothermal therapy denervate and repair experimentally induced posterolateral annular tears in an animal model? Spine; 28(23): 2602–2608.

15. **Pauza KJ, Howell S, Dreyfuss P, et al** (2004) A randomized, placebo controlled trial of intradiscal electrothermal therapy for the treatment of discogenic low back pain. *Spine J;* 4(1): 27–35.

16. **Freeman BJC, Fraser RD, Cain CMJ, et al** (2005) A randomized controlled trial of intradiscal electrothermal therapy versus placebo for the treatment of chronic discogenic low back pain. *Spine* [In Press].

17. **Adams CI, Freeman BJC, Clark A, et al** (2005) Outcome of targeted foraminal epidural steroid injection for radicular pain: A Kaplan Meier survival analysis. *J Bone J Surg (Br);* Orth Proceedings Suppl III; 87-B:243.

18. **Aylott CEW, Leung YL, Freeman BJC, et al** (2005) Acute Biomechanical effects of a novel intradiscal decompression catheter on human lumbar discs. *J Bone J Surg (Br);* Orth Proceedings Suppl III; 87-B:37.

19. **Deen HG, Fenton D** (2004) Electrothermal disc decompression: preliminary experience. *Presented at IITS meeting,* Munich, Germany: May 19–24.

2.8   GENERAL TECHNIQUES OF SPINAL DECOMPRESSION

1   INTRODUCTION

Neural decompressive procedures are the most commonly performed spinal operations. The procedures have remained largely unchanged over the past few decades; however, they have been refined with the introduction of better imaging and microsurgical techniques. The importance of history and physical examination cannot be overemphasized to make an appropriate diagnosis and to localize the level clinically before imaging is requested. The purpose of this chapter is to describe the decompressive procedures involving the cervical, thoracic, and lumbar spine.

2   UPPER CERVICAL AND CRANIOCERVICAL DECOMPRESSION

Anterior approaches

The transoral-transpharyngeal route is used to access pathology located in the anterior extradural area located from the lower clivus to the upper cervical spine [1, 2]. The patient is positioned supine on the operating table. Fiber-optic endoscopy is used in cases of anticipated difficult intubation. The head is immobilized. The oral cavity is prepared, retractors are positioned, and the operating microscope introduced. After obtaining a lateral x-ray, the posterior pharyngeal wall is incised. With the help of subperiosteal dissection, self-retaining retractors are placed to expose the clivus, C1, and C2. The decompression is performed with a combination of a high-speed drill, curettes, and rongeurs.

Lateral approaches

The patient is positioned laterally on the operating table. The far lateral approach is undertaken by making a skin incision extending from the midline to the inion and then across to the mastoid tip. Again with the help of subperiosteal dissection, the suboccipital bone is exposed as well as the arch of C1. A suboccipital craniectomy is performed and the arch of C1 is removed to allow decompression of the neural elements.

Posterior approach

The patient is positioned prone on the operating table and the neck is flexed depending on the stability. A midline incision is made from the inion down to C3. A subperiosteal dissection is performed to expose the foramen magnum and C1 region. The bony removal is carried out with the help of a high-speed drill at the foramen magnum and a C1 laminectomy is performed. The dura may or may not be opened depending on the indication for the operation (**Fig 2.8-1**).

2.1   ANTERIOR CERVICAL DECOMPRESSION/DISCECTOMY AND FUSION

Anterior decompression of the subaxial spine is performed to either decompress the spinal cord (for a myelopathy) or the nerve roots (for a radiculopathy).

The patient is positioned supine with the neck slightly hyperextended with a sandbag between the shoulders and a chin-strap for traction. A right-sided transverse skin crease incision is made depending on the level of the pathology. A standard approach is used to access the anterior cervical spine.

It is imperative at this stage to stay in the midline. The longus colli muscles are identified on either side and undercut to allow the placement of retractor blades. Side-to-side as well as up-and-down retraction is used to expose the disc space(s). A plain x-ray is then taken with a needle marker to confirm the

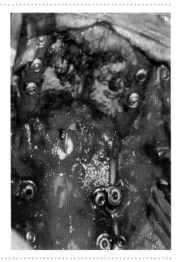

Fig 2.8-1
Posterior approach, occipitocervical fusion, and decompression.

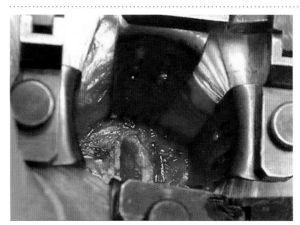

Fig 2.8-2
After discectomy.

level. The disc is then incised with a scalpel blade and removed with the help of pituitary rongeurs (**Fig 2.8-2**). The operating microscope is introduced and the osteophyte is removed with a high-speed drill or with fine Kerrison punches. The disc is removed until the posterior longitudinal ligament is exposed. The posterior longitudinal ligament is opened to thoroughly decompress the dura. The exiting nerve root is decompressed out laterally. An autogenous iliac crest bone graft or cage implant may be placed in the disc space followed by application of an anterior cervical plate.

The potential complications of this procedure include:

- injury to the larynx and trachea,
- injury to the esophagus and pharynx,
- injury to the recurrent laryngeal nerve,
- injury to the carotid sheath,
- injury to the vertebral artery,
- injury to the sympathetic chain,
- increasing neurological deficit,
- dural laceration and CSF (cerebrospinal fluid) fistula,
- graft extrusion, migration, and pseudarthrosis,
- screw loosening and pullout.

2.2   POSTERIOR CERVICAL DECOMPRESSION

Decompression of the cervical spine can be performed posteriorly and this has some advantages. The posterior approach is technically less challenging; it does not usually require additional instrumentation/bone grafting, and the posterior route does not stiffen the motion segments. If multilevel decompression is performed then instrumentation is applied (**Fig 2.8-3**).

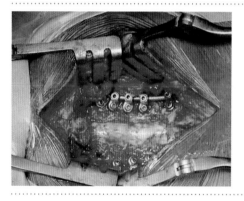

Fig 2.8-3
Decompression and fusion for stability.

Cervical laminectomy

This procedure is performed with the patient positioned prone on the operating table, with the head immobilized usually with three-point head fixation (Mayfield head clamp), or with the head simply supported in a horseshoe head ring. A midline incision is made, and sharp and blunt subperiosteal dissection allows exposure of the posterior spinal elements (**Fig 2.8-4a**). A plain x-ray is taken to confirm the levels, following which the dural sac is decompressed. This is either done with the help of bone nibblers and Kerrison punches or a high-speed drill. The spinous processes and the laminae are removed—great care must be taken when inserting the Kerrison punches as any degree of force may lead to neurological injury. The ligamentum flavum is incised and opened and then removed to visualize and decompress the dura (**Fig 2.8-4b**).

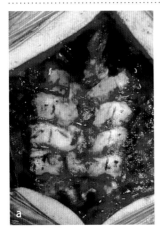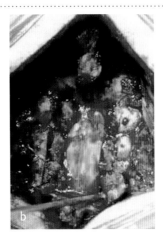

Fig 2.8-4a–b
a Spine exposed and marked ready to do the laminectomy.
b Laminectomy completed.

Cervical foraminotomy

Again the patient is placed prone and the head fixed or supported. In the case of bony cervical nerve root compression and occasionally with a laterally placed disc herniation, a foraminotomy can be performed. This procedure involves decompression of the hemilamina and removing the inferior margin of the superior lamina, which allows visualization of the nerve root. This procedure can also be chosen instead of the anterior approach for a disc prolapse in patients who depend upon their voice for a living, as anterior cervical surgery carries the small risk of injury to the recurrent laryngeal nerve and thus the patient may suffer hoarseness of voice as a result.

Cervical laminoplasty

Patient position and exposure is carried out as for a cervical laminectomy. A laminoplasty requires detaching one side of the lamina from the facet while leaving the other side intact. The high-speed drill is used to create a trough bilaterally and the small Kerrison punches used on the side of the pathology to detach the lamina from the facet. Hence, a door is created which, when opened, decompresses the spinal cord. The nerve roots are decompressed on the open side. Once the decompression is completed, the door is closed and small low-profile plates are applied between the lamina and the facet joints.

Any of these posterior cervical procedures, particularly laminectomy, carry the risk of creating spinal instability. If there is any concern about stability, consideration should be given to posterior cervical instrumentation. Laminoplasty is recommended for younger patients with benign pathology.

3   THORACIC DISCECTOMY

Disc herniation is much less common in the thoracic spine compared to the cervical and lumbar spine. Thoracic disc herniation is often asymptomatic, and the indication for surgery is either severe unremitting radicular pain in the chest wall or a progressive myelopathy.

There are various approaches described depending on:

- the level of the disc prolapse,
- laterality of the disc,
- calcification,
- the patient's general medical condition.

Posterior approaches
- laminectomy and transpedicular approach.

Lateral approaches
- costotransversectomy and extracavitary approach.

Ventrolateral approaches
- transthoracic thoracotomy,
- retropleural approach,
- anterior transternal approach.

For the purpose of this chapter, the transthoracic thoracotomy approach is described as this is possibly the most commonly performed approach for symptomatic thoracic disc herniation.

The patient is intubated and ventilated with a double lumen endotracheal tube to allow selective collapse of one lung. Usually, for disc herniations at the middle and lower parts of the thoracic spine, a left-sided approach is employed to minimize injury to the inferior vena cava. The patient is positioned in the lateral position. A preoperative marker plain x-ray can be useful in identifying the level of the disc to be resected.

A skin incision is made over the rib. The subcutaneous tissue is incised and the thoracic muscles are cut with diathermy down to the rib. The periosteum is then elevated, the rib is incised, and the parietal pleura opened. The lung at this stage is collapsed by the anesthetist and is retracted. The segmental vessels need to be ligated and divided. The sympathetic chain is preserved. A repeat plain x-ray is performed to confirm the level. The head of the rib is then removed. The pedicle of the vertebra is removed and the adjacent parts of the vertebral bodies are excised with a high-speed drill. The herniated disc is then delivered anteriorly and removed.

Hemostasis is very carefully secured before closure. If there is any concern regarding stability, autogenous graft from the earlier resected rib is replaced, and interbody fusion with plate/rod and screws is undertaken. A chest drain is inserted postoperatively to reestablish negative pressure and lung expansion.

3.1 COMPLICATIONS

Approach related complications:

- pneumothorax,
- pneumonia,
- atelectasis,
- hemothorax,
- rarely, bronchopleural fistulas.

General complications:

- infection, especially of the chest,
- death.

Spinal cord complications:

- neurological deficit with paralysis,
- CSF leak.

3.2 THORACIC DECOMPRESSION

Thoracic decompression for degenerative disease is rarely indicated but malignancy or infection may require such an approach. If a posterior thoracic decompression is required it is performed as in the cervical spine and again combined with posterior stabilization if required.

4 LUMBAR DISCECTOMY

The most important factor predicting outcome in lumbar disc surgery is patient selection. As highlighted earlier, a good history and neurological examination is essential for deciding clinically the relevant level of disc protrusion before imaging is requested. The primary aim of lumbar discectomy is to relieve leg pain, as removal of a prolapsed lumbar disc is not indicated for predominant back pain.

4.1 PROCEDURE

The most common patient position is the knee-chest position, but this procedure can also be performed with the patient in the prone position or lateral position. It is imperative to check the abdomen is free to prevent venous engorgement.

A preoperative needle marker plain x-ray is obtained especially if a small incision is contemplated. A midline incision is made and dissection is carried down to open the lumbar fascia. A subperiosteal dissection is then carried out to place the retractors and expose the relevant laminae. Removing the inferior edge of the superior lamina can then widen the interspace. The ligamentum flavum is then opened and removed to complete the fenestration.

The thecal sac and the nerve root are then identified. These structures are usually covered with epidural fat. If at all possible, one should not attempt to remove the epidural fat from the dura. This may be important to prevent future scar formation around the nerve root and also minimizes epidural bleeding at this stage of the operation. The fenestration should be carried laterally to prevent excessive retraction on the nerve root while removing the disc fragments (**Fig 2.8-5**).

The nerve root is then retracted medially to remove the prolapsed disc fragments. If the preoperative imaging is suggestive of a free disc fragment, it can be delivered with ease by elevating the nerve root gently. If the disc fragment is contained with an intact annulus fibrosus, the blade is used to make an incision in the annulus. The pituitary rongeurs are then inserted into the disc space to remove the degenerate disc material. A blunt hook and curettes can also be used to excise disc material. The ultimate aim of the operation is decompression of the nerve root. Once the root becomes slack and adequate amounts of disc material have been removed, one should stop, as aggressive curettage of the end plates bears no advantage in terms of outcome. The primary object is to make sure that the disc space is cleared, the subligamentous area beneath the nerve root is cleared, and both cranial and caudal exploration has been performed to look for any free fragments.

Management of a CSF leak

If a CSF leak occurs, an attempt at primary closure is recommended. However, if the durotomy is laterally placed, then it is appropriate to place a cottonoid patty over the leak and continue the removal of the disc. If a primary closure is not pos-

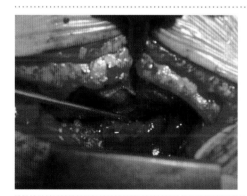

Fig 2.8-5
Lumbar discectomy.

sible, a muscle-and-fat graft is placed together with tissue glue. The patient is kept flat in bed for a period up to 48 hours.

Management of epidural bleeding

Epidural bleeding can be troublesome especially after removal of a large prolapsed disc. It generally responds to placement of patties and application of gentle pressure. It may require bipolar diathermy and, rarely, tissue glue and other hemostatic agents.

Steps to prevent surgery at the wrong level

One of the reasons for a poor result is surgery at the wrong level. A preoperative plain x-ray with a needle marker should be obtained. A repeat plain film can be performed before fenestration of the ligamentum flavum and a final plain x-ray should be taken with an instrument in the disc space at the end of the discectomy.

4.2   COMPLICATIONS

- Superficial wound infection,
- deep seated infection,
- dural tear resulting in CSF leak and infection requiring further surgery,
- nerve root damage,
- cauda equina syndrome,
- recurrent/residual disc prolapse,
- injury of retroperitoneal structures such as bowel and major vessels (rare).

4.3   LUMBAR SPINE DECOMPRESSION

Lumbar spine decompression is usually carried out for neurogenic claudication, ie, pain in the legs when walking. This has to be differentiated from intermittent claudication which is due to vascular insufficiency, where the peripheral pulses are often absent. Classically, a patient with neurogenic claudication will complain of pain on walking a certain distance. At the onset of pain, they will stop and bend forward in order to gain relief after which they will resume walking. Lumbar spine stenosis is classified into central canal stenosis and lateral recess stenosis.

Procedure

The patient is positioned prone on the operating table on rolls/wedges. A midline incision is made to cover the area of decompression. After incising the lumbar fascia, bilateral muscle stripping is done with blunt and sharp dissection. The facet joints are preserved. A plain x-ray is performed to confirm the levels of decompression. The spinous processes are removed and a laminectomy is carried out. The laminae are removed bilaterally to expose the ligamentum flavum. The ligamentum flavum is removed with Kerrison punches to expose the dura (**Fig 2.8-6**). The nerve roots are decompressed by undercutting the facet joints. It is essential to decompress the nerves by removing the ligamentum flavum, and great care should be taken when decompressing nerve roots as CSF leak can result if the dura is caught in the Kerrison punches.

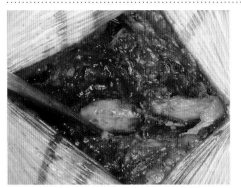

Fig 2.8-6
Lumbar laminectomy with decompression of the dura.

5 SUGGESTIONS FOR FURTHER READING

Benzel EC (1999) *Spine Surgery: Techniques, Complication Avoidance, and Management.* 2nd ed. London: Churchill Livingstone.

Crockard A, Hayward R, Hoff JT (2000) *Neurosurgery: The Scientific Basis of Clinical Practice.* 3rd ed. Oxford: Blackwell Science.

Dickman CA, Spetzler RF, Sonntag VK (1998) *Surgery of the Craniovertebral Junction.* 1st ed. New York: Thieme Medical Publishers.

Schmidek HH, Sweet WH (1995) *Operative Neurosurgical Techniques: Indications, Methods and Results.* 4th ed. Philadelphia: WB Saunders Co.

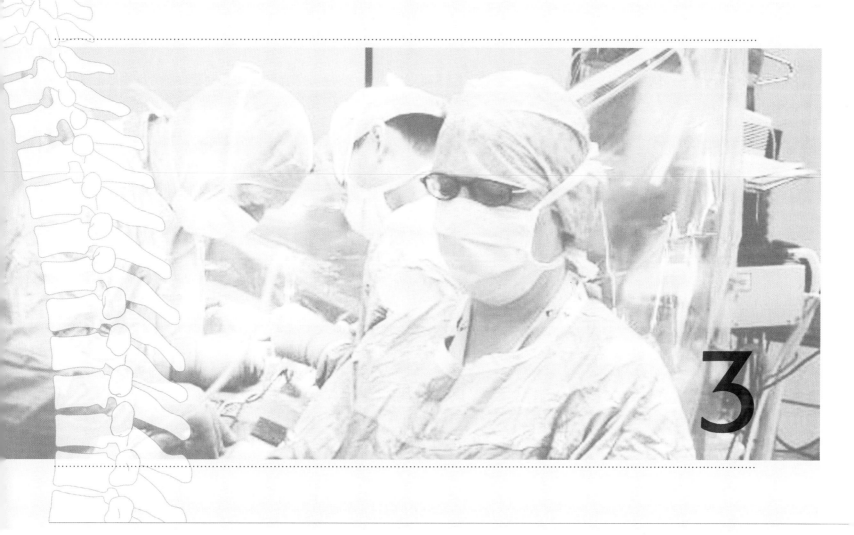

OPERATIVE KNOWLEDGE
FOR SPINE SURGERY

3

3   OPERATIVE KNOWLEDGE FOR SPINE SURGERY
3.1   INFECTION CONTROL AND PREVENTATIVE PRECAUTIONS IN THE OPERATING ROOM

3.1   INFECTION CONTROL AND PREVENTATIVE PRECAUTIONS IN THE OPERATING ROOM

1   INTRODUCTION

Healthcare staff are accountable to ensure the care they deliver is of the highest possible standard. Our role as operating room personnel (ORP) is to fulfill patient's needs while in our care, with the help of operating room (OR) users from other multidisciplinary healthcare teams. We complete a variety of duties during the course of the day to ensure organizational efficiency and clinical effectiveness within the operating suite, but none as important as risk management based around infection control.

2   RISK FACTORS

There are many risk factors to consider in relation to infection, with regard to the patient, surgery and the situation [1] in any surgical procedure, but in spine surgery the risk factors can increase as shown in **Table 3.1-1**.

Gourlay [2] lists other factors which may influence surgical wound infections within the OR suite, eg, ventilation and air filtration, sterility of instruments, and surgical scrub technique.

Patient	• age group—when very young/old
	• rheumatoid arthritis
	• size/weight—eg, obese
	• nutritional status
	• malignancy
	• acute infection prior to surgery
	• underlying diseases
	• renal failure
	• diabetic
	• blood transfusions
	• steroid/cytotoxic therapy
	• foreign bodies
Surgery	• surgical wound classification
	• emergency surgery
	• operative site
	• length of surgery
	• wound contamination during surgery
	• use of drains
	• surgical technique
	• wound closure
	• length of incision
	• implants in situ
Situation	• ultra clean OR—clean air systems, stringent cleaning at end of OR list
	• length of preoperative stay
	• presence of other infections
	• preoperative preparation
	• skin preparation
	• number of people in OR
	• traffic volume during the surgery

Table 3.1-1
Risk factors that impact on infection.

Patients who undergo surgery are immediately susceptible to wound infections, due to the break in their skin integrity and the insertion of instruments into body tissue [3]. Infection comes with a price tag; the cost element should not be taken out of the equation. This also comes at a price for the patient, for the following reasons:

- discomfort suffered,
- extended hospitalization for antibiotic therapy and care,
- anxiety/stress due to possible readmission,
- possible loss of earnings.

Stress can become a major factor with regard to infection. Stress is well documented as a cause that can prolong wound healing, recovery time and possibly cause death.

Important practices relating to infection control in the OR have been developed through research for many years in ORs worldwide. This information is especially important in relation to spine surgery, but should be practiced in all specialties.

3   PREVENTION OF INFECTION

The history of infection control in the OR began in the 19th century with the move from the ward to a designated area for surgical procedures. With this move, the OR was established in 1880 [4]. The prevention of infection requires many skills from ORP; they must be able to measure, map, and execute activities to ensure not only a clean OR suite but also a controlled aseptic surgical environment.

We must encourage healthcare practitioners to be responsible for putting guidelines into practice. Clarke and Jones [3] state: "We must consider up-to-date clinical research when operating department policies are written, to ensure that policies are based on research not ritual". To reduce the risk of infection we must be committed to a high standard of infection control practice for all patients in all care activities within the OR environment.

One practice which can be applied is house rules or surgical environmental guidelines. These are produced to encourage the entire surgical team to comply with the policies set. Below are suggested house rules.

All personnel before entering the OR:

- Ensure hair is completely covered by headwear.
- Masks must be worn if sterile trays are open (follow hospital policies).
- No jewelery to be worn (except wedding rings).
- Do not bring in personal bags or briefcases.
- Ensure OR dress/attire is clean.
- Ensure footwear is clean (overshoes are not acceptable).
- Perform a general hand wash prior to entry.

Circulating personnel and visitors:

- Do not enter/leave the OR without cause.
- Reduce traffic by keeping movement to a minimum.
- Do not enter the clean air enclosure unless essential to perform a task.
- Do not lean into the clean air enclosure for a better view.
- Do not use other scrub, preparation, anesthetic, or operating rooms as a shortcut or walkthrough if they are interconnected.

Scrub personnel/surgeons:

- Hair must be completely covered, regardless of headwear chosen.
- An approved method of scrubbing up must be used.
- An approved method must be used for donning gowns and gloves.
- Once gowned and gloved do not leave the clean air enclosure unless absolutely necessary.
- Discard gowns/gloves in the appropriate bags/containers immediately after use.

These house rules are intended specifically for the patient's benefit.

4   MICROORGANISMS

To address infection control we need to educate ourselves as to what we are dealing with. Human beings are said to be contaminated with microorganisms from birth [5]. Microorganisms are described as normal flora or commensals which live in harmony with the host, ie, a symbiotic relationship. When the host's defenses are breached, such as in surgery, they then become pathogenic, which leads to infection.

Spine surgery is seen as a high-risk area for endogenous or exogenous infections, due to the disruption of tissues and bone during surgery.

The main organisms relating to orthopedic surgery are:

- *Staphylococcus aureus*–wound sepsis which includes methicillin-resistant *Staphylococcus aureus* (MRSA),
- *Staphylococcus epidermidis*–infected bone,
- diphtheroids–implant involvement,
- gram-negative bacilli–osteomyelitis.

Sadly, in addition to the above, the modern healthcare environment has developed a major by-product associated with treating inpatients with hospital aquired infections (HAIs). The bacteria is found in the hospital setting and associated with infected equipment, staff, and patients. This is an unfortunate side effect of treating large numbers of people in close proximity [6]. The principal documented causes of HAIs are the result of microbial contamination of the wound during surgery.

First detected in the 1960s, methicillin-resistant *Staphylococcus aureus* is the most well-publicized HAI. Also known as the "superbug" of bacteria, MRSA has occurred due to the overprescribing of antibiotics over many years. It lives harmlessly on the skin and in the nose of 30% of the population of the United Kingdom [6]. However, in some cases it can have a dramatic effect on patients who have had surgery, when the bacteria invade the wound. It can develop from an insignificant infection to a life-threatening condition.

The source of MRSA colonization has been well documented; via their hands, healthcare workers are unfortunately the primary transmitters of the bacteria. The surgical team can reduce this risk by following stringent infection control procedures in the OR.

There are other environmental aspects of preventing infection but the most important is general hand hygiene both on the ward and in the OR. However, we do need to take into consideration other factors associated with surgery:

- Preparation of the scrub team—it has been well published that hand hygiene is a fundamental factor in addressing HAI, so scrubbing, gowning, and glove donning technique practices should be of the highest standard.
- The carrier—skin.
- Bathing and showering.
- Shaving and clipping.
- Patient skin preparation and sterile draping to establish a sterile field— the combination of appropriate skin preparation and disposable drapes aim to reduce the risk of postoperative infections.
- Postoperative wound closure—suturing and skin clips.
- Postoperative drainage systems.
- Central venous lines.
- Wound dressings.

All of these practices are the responsibility of the entire surgical team (the powerful) in order to protect the patient (the powerless) during surgical procedures.

5   KEY POINTS FOR THE SCRUB TEAM

Scrubbing up

Performing a surgical scrub prior to donning a sterile gown and gloves will not leave your hands and arms sterile, but will reduce the amount of microorganisms on the skin. This is to reduce the risk of contamination to the patient if the surgical glove is perforated at any time during the procedure.

All ORs/suites should hold their own up-to-date scrubbing policies and all members of the scrub team must comply.

The main points to follow when scrubbing are:

- Team members with upper respiratory infections, broken skin areas on hands or arms must not scrub.
- No jewellery should be worn.
- Hair and face covered correctly with hat and mask.
- Nonscrub OR attire should feel comfortable.
- The finger nails should be clean and short with no false or polished nails prior to scrubbing. Scrub brushes should only be used on nails for the first scrub of the day, as these can cause micro-abrasions to the skin.
- Water temperature should be set at a comfortable level.
- Use solutions recommended for surgical scrubs that are non ethanol-based products.
- 5 ml of solution to be used for application, worked into hands and arms before rinsing—three applications recommended in total.
- A 2 minute scrub is suggested—3 minutes is more ideal.
- At all times during scrubbing hands must be held above elbows to prevent scrub solutions/water revisiting the clean region.
- Rinsing is performed from fingers to elbow, and never the reverse.

- A separate sterile towel must be used for each hand. Hands should be dried using a dabbing technique rather than rubbing as this will reduce the risk of skin problems.
- Once scrubbed the hands must be kept above the elbows (**Fig 3.1-1a–d**).

Gowning up

Donning a sterile gown provides a protective barrier between the patient and the staff member, preventing cross contamina-

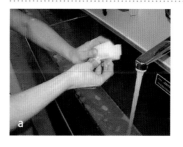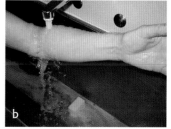
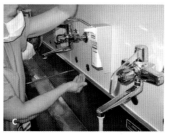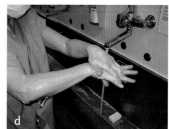

Fig 3.1-1a–d
a Using a scrub brush.
b Always run water from hand to elbow.
c Dispensing scrub solution.
d Washing between fingers.

tion from patient to staff and vice versa. The type and style used will depend on hospital budgets and supplier, but the key points are:

- Gowns must be in a good state of repair.
- Gowns must be nonpermeable and be able to wrap fully around the scrub member.
- When donning, the scrub member should only touch the inside of the gown.
- The circulating personnel should tie the gown at the neck and waist only.
- Hands should never be passed through the cuff; closed technique for donning gloves should be performed.
- If contamination occurs at any stage while donning, the gown must be discarded and replaced.
- The gown should only be touched with sterile gloved hands (**Fig 3.1-2a–d**).

Glove donning
The gloves used are the individual team member's preference. There are many types and styles available in today's market and the individual scrub member should find one that is comfortable for them. Latex allergies are increasing in healthcare, particularly in relation to glove use. This can have a dramatic affect on both patient and team member if the risk has not been highlighted prior to surgery. Therefore, it is crucial that the patient is asked for all known allergies, including latex, before the anesthetic is administered.

- The closed-glove-donning method is preferred (**Fig 3.1-3a–h, Fig 3.1-4a–b**). The scrub personnel assist the remaining team members with glove donning.
- Wear gloves that are comfortable, both in the fingers and round the cuff.

- Do not wear gloves that feel tight; this can cause the wearer circulation problems in the fingers during the surgery.
- In spine surgery always double glove for your own protection, especially in relation to needle-stick injury and sharp bone perforation.
- Wear an indicator glove as the first pair. Thus, any perforation not seen under normal circumstances will be highlighted during the surgery [1, 3].

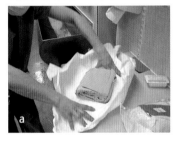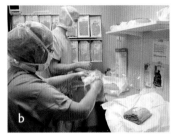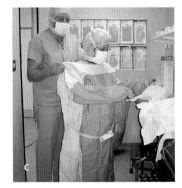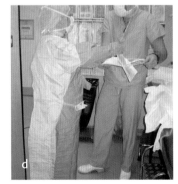

Fig 3.1-2a–d
a   Preparing to gown up.
b–d Gowning up and receiving gloves.

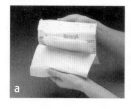

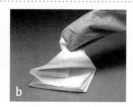

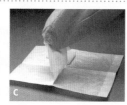

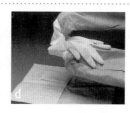

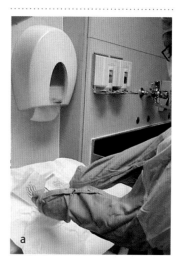

1. Open the pack from the corners and gently peel from the top of the pack, rolling hands and wrists outwards as if opening a book.

2. Open inner pack, so that the right glove is directly opposite the right hand. The forceps flap may be used if desired.

3. Through the gown, grasp the cuff of the left glove with the right hand and remove the glove from the pack.

4. Place the glove on the left wrist. Through the gown, grasp the lower cuff edge with the left thumb. Grasp the top of the glove with right thumb under the cuff edge. While still gripping the glove, make a fist.

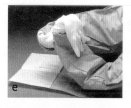

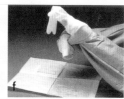

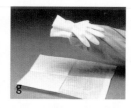

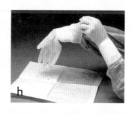

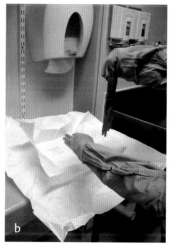

5. Stretch the cuff over the hand aiming to cover the knuckles and thumb joint before straightening the fingers on the right hand.

6. Pull the sleeve of the sterile gown with the protected hand, keeping the fingers of the right hand straight so the glove can easily be pulled into place.

7. The gloved left hand now picks up the right glove. As before, place the glove on the wrist.

8. Make a fist and pull the glove over the gown and maneuver to give a good fit. The gloves can now be adjusted without fear of contamination.

Fig 3.1-3a–h
The closed-glove-donning technique (reproduced with kind permission of Ansell UK LTD).

Fig 3.1-4a–b
Closed method for donning technique.

6   THE CARRIER—SKIN

What is skin? The skin consists of two layers, the epidermis and the dermis, and is the largest organ of the body. It measures about 1.5–2 mm in adults and weighs about 15% of total body weight [7].

The epidermis is the outer surface of the organ, with no blood vessels, glands, or nerve endings. It does, however, contain pigment, which gives the skin color, and pores to excrete sweat from the glands in the dermis.

The dermis is the inner elastic foundation which contains blood, lymphatic vessels, nerves, sweat glands, and hair follicles.

Together their function is to:

- hold and protect the contents of the body,
- excrete waste made up of 99% water and 1% salts,
- act as a thermostat controlling body temperature by maintaining a core temperature of 37°C,
- conserve heat in response to a drop in temperature,
- protect against ultraviolet light,
- protect against infections and chemicals—only if the skin sustains no trauma,
- act as a conductor for the body to receive stimuli against temperature changes and pain, allowing the brain to react to avoid damage.

7   PREOPERATIVE SKIN PREPARATION

The topic of shaving and preoperative bathing has been the subject of some discussion and research in the past, and its status remained unchallenged until the 1970s. At this time questions arose regarding its impact on postoperative wound infections [7].

7.1   BATHING AND SHOWERING

This was a practice encouraged on the ward for many years prior to OR, using antiseptic solutions. Byrne et al [10] implied that the patient would need to shower at least three times with chlorhexidine to effectively reduce the bacterial count.

Freshwater [11] looked at what the value and impact of preoperative bathing versus showering had prior to surgery. The cleanliness of baths between uses should also be addressed as a possible platform for the transfer of bacterial organisms.

Washing with soap and water removes soil and transient microorganisms from the surface of the skin. However, this mechanical debridement tends to expose resident flora, leading to an increase in surface bacteria counts.

7.2   SHAVING AND CLIPPING

Surgical site shaving was routine until challenged, when suggestions were made that it caused superficial damage to the skin, thus allowing bacterial colonization [8]. However, shaving is a prerequisite for some spine surgery procedures and may be undertaken when the patient is positioned. In many cases the thigh requires shaving to allow the diathermy plate to adhere to the skin as a point of contact.

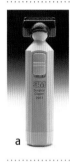
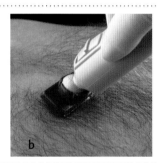

Fig 3.1-5a–b
Skin clipper
(reproduced with
kind permission of
3M Health Care
Limited).

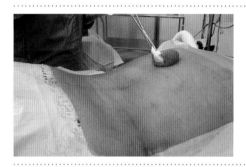

Fig 3.1-6
Skin prepping.

Clipping is the recommended way of removing hair prior to surgery; shaving should only be carried out if hair removal cannot be achieved by depilatory cream the day before surgery, or in the anesthetic room using clippers (**Fig 3.1-5a–b**) instead of razors. Three recommendations with regard to shaving/clipping are shown below [9]:

- Avoid shaving if at all possible.
- Use depilatory cream. If this is not possible, use clippers.
- Only shave if other options are not possible.

7.3   SKIN PREPARATION

This procedure is performed once the multidisciplinary team has agreed that the patient has been positioned correctly, and all the positioning risks have been addressed in preparation for the surgery about to commence.

Preparation of the patient's skin for surgery has been addressed time and time again. Various methods of preprepping prior to

surgery have been adopted over the years. One method commonplace on the orthopedic wards both witnessed and practiced by the author 30 years ago, was preprepping on the ward by painting the limb with a disinfectant and wrapping the limb in linen prior to the OR. Some teams moved on to prepping in the anesthetic room and again on the operating table. The spinal patient cannot be prepprepped due to positioning, so the patient can only be prepped on the table, this is performed twice before draping, allowing drying time in between each application.

Applying an antibacterial skin preparation to the patient's operative site reduces the surface bacteria to subpathogenic levels over a short period of time. This also inhibits a rapid rebound growth of microorganisms, with the least amount of tissue disruption and irritation possible.

Regardless of the solution chosen, the incision site plus a generous surrounding area must be thoroughly prepared (**Fig 3.1-6**). Cleansing begins at the proposed incision site and continues laterally towards the perimeter of the patient's skin, never returning to the proposed incision site.

7.4   COMMON SOLUTIONS

Common solutions are:

- iodine in alcohol,
- povidine iodine,
- cetrimide,
- chlorhexidine.

While each solution has advantages and disadvantages, iodine or chlorhexidine are generally the preferred solutions for spine surgery and are very effective in reducing the number of bacteria present on the intact skin. It is very important that the solution used is allowed to dry naturally on the patient's skin especially if linen drapes are used. Linen drapes, when wet, can contaminate nonprepared areas of skin (see 8 Draping, in this chapter). Excessive use which leads to pooling of the solutions should also be avoided.

Povidine iodine
Scientific studies have shown povidine iodine to be very effective against microorganisms; including MRSA. The solution is also proven to be an active bactericidal against gram-positive staphylococcal and gram-negative pseudomonas.

In 1998 a skin preparation was introduced into the UK which contained 0.7% w/w available iodine and 74% w/w isopropyl alcohol. The indications for use were for a long-lasting preoperative preparation with a broad-spectrum antimicrobial activity. This was a unit dose, single step, and one applicator delivery. With superior resistance to removal by blood and saline it rapidly dried to give a nonsticky surface.

The author conducted a randomized, controlled, in-house trial for 100 patients using this new product within the spinal ORs (**Table 3.1-2**).

The two skin preparations in the trial:

- new product—50 patients,
- iodine in alcohol—50 patients.

Patient criteria:

- primary surgery at the surgical site,
- lumbar surgery only.

At the time the trial took place the postoperative infection rate was approximately 4%.

Formula for trial	New product	Alcoholic iodine
Ease of use	95%	5%
Application control	90%	10%
Drying comparison	91%	9%
Allergic reaction	0%	0%
Adhesion during surgery	95%	5%

Table 3.1-2
New product: trial results.

Postoperative results showed that only four patients returned with superficial or deep wound infections—three in the iodine in alcohol arm and one in the new product arm of the study.

Alcoholic iodine: 1 × MRSA and 2 × staphylococcus aureus, all three patients returned between 1–2 months postoperative. New product: 1 × superficial wound leakage, no growth found, returned 5 months postoperative.

It was on these results that the new product was introduced, as the preferred skin preparation of choice in 2001. We experienced a dramatic reduction in postoperative wound infections during the 3 years this product was in use.

Sadly, the company who supplied this product ceased sales activity in the UK in 2005, but it is available elsewhere in Europe and the USA.

Dating back to 1981 there have been calls for recommended single-dose measures of skin disinfects. Yet almost 25 years later multipour containers, which are a potential source of infection once opened to the natural elements, are still in general use. The practice of "topping up" is no doubt a temptation given budgetary constraints, but this practice must not occur given the potential for contamination. The new product did meet the demands of a single-use skin preparation. The cost of a single infection would make it more cost effective to open multiuse bottles and discard them after single patient use; this however only increases the manufacturer's profit margins [3].

The type of skin preparation used may vary, but the end result should be:

- Disinfection of the skin.
- Continual effectiveness of solution throughout the surgery.
- Complete adhesion of the drape to the patient's skin, as disturbance of the drapes will contaminate the surgical field with unwanted microorganisms.

8   DRAPING

Draping is an essential phase of the surgical procedure. The aim is to achieve a sterile surgical field prior to the surgical incision by optimal barrier performance of the drape. This is a vital role in prevention of contamination of the surgical site, and must not be breached with nonsterile items during the procedure.

A surgical drape is a sterilized piece of material—linen, reusable barrier, disposable, or plastic. The aim of the drape is to provide an efficient barrier between a sterile and nonsterile area. Linen drapes have been the drape of choice within the OR for many years. Amongst some surgeons linen is still the preferred drape, mainly because of its flexibility and how it envelopes the limbs. Davidson [12] highlighted the fact that linen and disposables can both be seen within some surgical fields. Disposables have the advantage of an adhesive edge with which to gain total isolation of the wound (**Fig 3.1-7a–c**).

Many surveys on disposable versus linen or barrier drapes have been conducted over the years. One of the main issues highlighted is the suggestion that disposables are more expensive.

Factors which could prevent use of disposable drapes are:

- purchase price,
- storage space expenditure,
- disposable expenditure,
- environmental cost.

Suggesting that a disposable drape is more expensive is very shortsighted; treating patients with postoperative infections would certainly offset any draping costs. A general consensus within the OR is that linen drapes should be removed completely and disposables introduced across the board. However, cost is seen as an issue in preventing a total change.

Multiple patient use (MPU) drapes made of muslin provide little protection against bacteria migrating from a nonsterile surface to a sterile surface. Once linen materials become soiled or wet, microorganisms can be carried through the drapes by a wicking action.

Fig 3.1-7a–c
a Disposable spine drapes—operative site squared off.
b Disposable all in one operative drape—patient positioned supine.
c Disposable all in one operative drape—patient positioned prone.

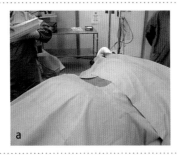
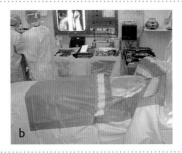
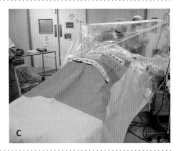

The cost/expenditure aspects involved for using MPU drapes are:

- Capital purchase cost—linen, autoclaves (which require maintenance).
- Repair costs—including sewing room staff, cottons, patch materials.
- Cleaning costs—washing machines, detergents, hot water.
- Ironing costs—irons, iron boards, presses.
- Staffing costs.
- Sterilization process—paper, microbial indicators, heat indicators, tape.
- Electrical energy costs.
- Cost of the employers health and safety aspects relating to all processes, insurance, training and sickness benefit in the case of an accident.
- Infection risk costs.
- Protocol/policy costs —setting and updating.

Environmental issues

There is significant concern regarding the disposal of single patient use (SPU) and MPU drapes. We should question what effect this may have on our environment, both now and in the future.

In 2000, the author's hospital—with a total of 1,200 beds—showed that the volume of clinical waste disposal was 685 tons per year, with a cost of £260 (USD 450) per ton; an annual cost of £178,000 (USD 310,000). The ORs are said to have the highest clinical waste volume within a hospital, the national average of waste having been calculated at 3 kg per hospital bed per day.

Bell [13] states in 1998: "The majority of manufacturers of SPU devices manufacture them to strict guidelines, most packaging is also made from recycled products and within 5 years the United Kingdom must come into line with other European countries that are required by law to reclaim a percentage of their waste products and recycle them." So why are MPU products still in use in 2005? The cleaning and sterilizing of MPU products have their own environmental implications, requiring energy and further resources, eg, packaging, which also creates waste. Thus it should not automatically be assumed that MPU products are more environmentally friendly.

A study was conducted on current surgical practices in 2003 investigating factors which influence the decision to use linen or disposable drapes. The results are shown below in **Table 3.1-3**. The draping systems were marked out of 10 (10 being the highest and 0 being the lowest). The results show disposable drapes as being superior in controlling infection [12].

Factor	Linen drapes	Disposable drapes
Infection control	4	10
Ease of handling	8	8
Cost effectiveness	7	8
Absorbency	5	8
Strikethrough	4	9
Regulations	4	10
Environmental costs	6	8
Health and safety of staff	5	10

Table 3.1-3
Rating of draping systems (10 = high, 0 = low).

In 2003 a document was accepted, although not at the time published, to establish uniform standards for single-use and reusable surgical drapes and gowns. It was designed to reduce the spread of bacteria and other microorganisms during invasive surgery to prevent postoperative wound infections. So the new European standard EN 13795 will be published in five parts:

• Part one—covers "general requirements for manufacturers, processors and products".
• Part two—test methods.
• Part three—test method for resistance to dry microbial penetration.
• Part four—test method for resistance to wet microbial penetration.
• Part five—performance requirements and performance levels.

This standard deals specifically with the prevention of infection in the OR [14]. This will no doubt force the practices of OR draping to change in the future. It has already been highlighted that linen drapes should not be recommended.

Historically the practice of prepping and draping in the OR was always seen as a surgeon's role. Taylor and Campbell [3] highlight that it is still the surgeon's ultimate responsibility. Both nurses and ORPs are or have been, quite happy to comply with the wishes of the surgeon, without question. This is not always the case today. In some areas nurses and ORPs will now challenge both care and practices within the work force.

The choice as to what drapes are used is a managerial decision made in conjunction with sisters/charge nurses/team leaders and the surgeon. At present, however, patients have no say regarding how they are draped during their surgical procedure. Given the ever-changing issues within the healthcare field, in the future patients may eventually have their say with regard to all aspects of their OR care, including their choice of draping and prepping methods.

Over the years concerns over SPU drapes versus MPU drapes are evident in nursing publications. The arguments for and against are documented time and time again, with SPU coming out as preferred by patients, nurses, ORP, and surgeons alike. Davidson [12] conducted a national survey in 2003 which reinforced what Bell [13] showed in 1998.

It has been acknowledged within the author's OR by the staff in general, that disposable drapes are superior to linen drapes. As a professional workforce we must be doing all within our remit to reduce the risk to the patient and prevent microbial contamination of the wound during the patient's pathway through the OR.

9   POSTOPERATIVE WOUND CLOSURE

"A surgical wound is a major break in the patient's skin integrity and hence a possible entry route for pathogenic organisms" [3]. When addressing wound closure we must thus look at the whole picture, and consider what specific precautions/procedures must be carried out to ensure that the patient does not develop a postoperative infection.

Following surgery it is vital that the surgical wound is cleansed thoroughly before closure commences, as an infection in the wound can slow down the healing process. The best cleaning solution for wounds, by general consensus in the literature, is 0.9% sodium chloride. For best irrigation results the solution should irrigate the wound under some pressure. The surgical team must protect their eyes with goggles or visors during this procedure. Any hematoma or dead or dying tissue must be excised before closure as this can increase the potential for postoperative infection. The aim of any wound closure is to join only clean, healthy tissue together to optimize the healing process. Encouraging the practitioner to reducing tissue handling on the skin edges during closure is important in limiting epidermis and dermis damage. Firm suturing of each layer will minimize scarring and prevent poor wound closure, so as to reduce the possible introduction of microorganisms postoperatively.

Suturing
Suturing has been practiced for at least 4,000 years and remains the most common method of wound closure. There is a wide range of sutures available for all layers of a wound. Selecting the most appropriate suture material will achieve the best outcome. In spine surgery there are three layers associated with a spine wound (posterior being the most common wound): deep (muscle fascia), superficial (fat), and skin (dermis). If the wound is not sutured correctly, either too loosely or too tightly, the tissues can become damaged or devitalized.

The consequences may be delayed wound healing, an uneven scar line, and colonization of bacteria, which could result in further visits to the OR for surgical wound washouts. Sutures should be removed between 5–10 days postoperatively, once wound healing has occurred.

In some spine surgery skin clips (staples) are the preferred method for closing the dermis. These offer the same cosmetic results as sutures, but are a much faster method for closing wounds, and are believed to have a better resistance to infection than sutures. However, the cost is greater than for sutures, and this may be a factor to consider when deciding on the method for wound closure.

Wound drains
Most spine surgery will require prophylactic wound drainage postoperatively in order to avoid colonization of microbes from waste fluid sitting in the cavity created during the surgery. There are two types of drainage systems used in spine surgery.

- Passive drainage, also known as an open drainage system, which works with gravity. This is required to be placed at the distal end of the wound where the bodily fluids will collect. This will be used when there is a leakage of cerebrospinal fluid (CSF) postsurgery, as this will allow slow drainage of the CSF leaking into the wound until the dura heals.
- Active suction, or closed drainage system, which works with a vacuum or negative pressure, and so can be placed more cranially if the surgeon wishes. The extraction of exudate that accumulates in the wound postoperatively can help to prevent the risk of postoperative infection. This also helps to encourage tissue granulation by closing down the dead space that has occurred (**Fig 3.1-8**).

Chest drains are used for all thoracic spine surgery. The patient will have a chest drain/under water seal drain in situ postoperatively to drain excessive blood and fluids, and to prevent the ingress of air into the chest cavity (**Fig 3.1-9a–c**).

All drains are inserted aseptically into the wound after irrigation and prior to suturing the dermis. While the chest drain will always be sutured in place, the two other drains (passive/active) may or may not be sutured in place, depending on the preference of the surgeon.

Problems that can occur with drainage systems are:

- potential route for infection,
- removal by the patient if young or confused,
- accidental pull out during transfer from operating table to bed/trolley,
- blockage due to hematoma or excessive tissue deposits.

One major complication which can occur postoperatively following anterior cervical surgery is the drain becoming dislodged or pulled out. This type of surgery is high risk if the patient develops a hematoma. Pressure within the wound may cause respiratory dyspnea, and may even lead to respiratory

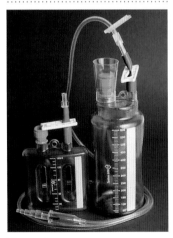

Fig 3.1-8
Medinorm drain (reproduced with kind permission of Summit Medical PLC).

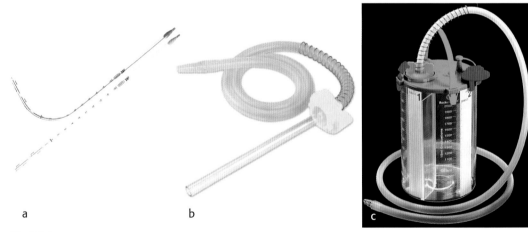

Fig 3.1-9a–c
a 28FG chest drain (reproduced with kind permission from Smith-Medical International LTD).
b Tube set (reproduced with kind permission of Rocket Medical PLC).
c Double chest drainage system.

arrest. The drain must always be sutured in place and the skin closed with staples to allow the release of the wound in the event of any sudden swelling.

Postoperatively, it is vitally important that staple removers remain in close proximity to the patient at all times as the onset of swift and unexpected swelling can cause serious and life-threatening complications for the patient.

Central venous lines

A central venous line (**Fig 3.1-10**) is a routine procedure used by the anesthetist in spine surgery. This catheter is fed through the jugular, subclavian or femoral veins into the superior vena cava or right atrium, to measure the patient's status relating to circulating fluid volume. This will help the anesthetist to decide throughout the surgery what fluid and blood products the patient requires. It also allows the rapid administration of fluids if the need arises.

There are several reasons for this catheter to be used during spine surgery:

- Fast administration of intravenous fluids, eg, when blood loss is excessive during the surgery, normally from epidural bleeding or an osteotomy.
- Administration of drugs postoperatively, eg, antibiotic.
- To monitor central venous pressure, eg, normal CVP range is 3–10 mmHg (5–12 cmH$_2$0).
- To postoperatively monitor major spinal cases, eg, deformity surgery.

Catheters can contain up to four lumen ports. This is of benefit when fluids are required while the CVP can still be monitored. However, single lumen catheters should be used unless multiple ports are essential. This device does have advantages but the patient can also develop complications arising from its use:

- pneumothorax,
- arterial puncture,
- cardiac dysrhythmias,
- air embolism,
- infection.

The catheter must be introduced under strict aseptic technique, and when it has been successfully introduced an x-ray should be taken to ensure it is correctly positioned. This procedure must be carried out to rule out the complications above. It is a highly invasive procedure, but it plays an important part in the patient's interoperative and postoperative care, as well as aiding in diagnosis and treatment.

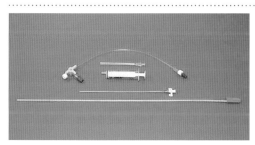

Fig 3.1-10
Central line (reproduced with kind permission from Vygon (UK) LTD).

Dressings

Dressings are applied to the wound for the following reasons:

- Protection of the wound surface and closures.
- Provision of a barrier against dirt and bacteria.
- Absorption of wound exudates.
- Promotion of the healing process by providing warmth and moisture.

There is now a superior knowledge of wound care and which style/type of dressing is required to promote healing. The vast range of dressings available for use is ever increasing, and quite radical. The type used immediately postoperatively in spine surgery is a mepore dressing which has the advantage of an adhesive backing, thus avoiding the use of tapes and bandages (**Fig 3.1-11a–c**).

For spine surgery the dressing must be adhesive due to the position of the majority of wounds. It is also advisable to place padding over the mepore dressing initially to absorb any exudates. This task can be performed either by the surgeon or the

ORP, but must be done as part of the surgical procedure under aseptic conditions. The surgical drapes must not be removed until the dressing has been secured on the wound, as this may cause cross contamination of the wound from the patients' own skin cells and microbes from other areas of the body.

This is seen as the final step and is an important part of the surgical procedure. Healing begins when the body temperature is at a normal 37°C. During surgery warming devices are used to maintain the patient's temperature, so it is important to cover the patient as soon as possible once the drapes have been removed in order to maintain the optimal temperature at which healing commences.

Removal or taking down of the dressing before the fourth day may interrupt the healing process and disturb granulation of the tissues. If the wound shows signs of heavy exudates the wound should be cleansed and redressed using an aseptic nontouch technique. Antibiotics may also be required; if so a swab of the wound should be sent to microbiology.

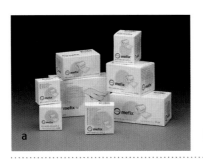 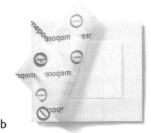 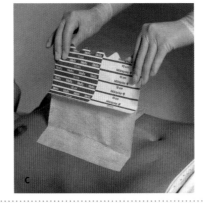

Fig 3.1-11a–c
A style of dressing suitable for spine surgery (reproduced with kind permission of Molnlycke Health Care Ltd).

10   BIBLIOGRAPHY

1. **Taylor M, Campbell C** (1999) Patient care in the operating department (2). *British Journal of Theatre Nursing;* 9(7):319–323.
2. **Gourlay D** (1994) Theatre practices. *Nursing Times;* 90(24): 64–68.
3. **Clarke P, Jones J** (1998) *Brigden's Operating Department Practice.* London: Churchill Livingston.
4. **Unerman E** (1994) Infection control in the operating department. *Surgical Nurse;* 7(1):31–34.
5. **Talaro KP, Talaro A** (1999) *Foundation in Microbiology.* 3rd ed. International edition. USA: McGraw–Hill.
6. **Beckford–Ball J, Hainsworth T** (2004) The control and prevention of hospital-acquired infections. *Nursing Times;* 100(29):28–29.
7. **Richardson M** (2003) Understanding the structure and function of the skin. *Nursing times Supp;* 99 (31):46–48.
8. **Woodhead K, Taylor EW, Bannister G,** et al (2002) Behaviors and rituals in the operating theatre. A report from the Hospital Infection Society Working Party on Infection Control in Operating Theatres. *J Hosp Infect;* 51(4):241–255.
9. **Seropian R, Reynolds BM** (1971) Wound infections after preoperative depilatory versus razor preparation. *Am J Surg;* 121(3):251–253.
10. **Byrne DJ, Phillips G, Napier A,** et al (1990) Rationalizing whole body disinfection. *J Hosp Infect;* 15(2):183–187.
11. **Freshwater D** (1992) Preoperative preparation of skin-a review of the literature. *Surgical Nurse,* 5(5):6–10.
12. **Davidson K, Dobb M, Tanner J** (2003) UK surgical draping practices. A national survey. *Br J Perioper Nurs;* 13(3):109–114.
13. **Bell S** (1998) Multiple patient use versus single patient use products. *British Journal of Theatre Nursing;* 8(1).
14. **NATN report from an Independent Multidisciplinary Working Group** (2003) *Considering The Consequences: an evaluation of infection risk when choosing surgical gowns and drapes in today's NHS.* February Ref No. 0012.

3   OPERATIVE KNOWLEDGE FOR SPINE SURGERY
3.2 ANESTHETICS AND ASSOCIATED COMPLICATIONS

3.2   ANESTHETICS AND ASSOCIATED COMPLICATIONS

1   INTRODUCTION

Provision of anesthesia for spine surgery is based on the fundamental principles covering anesthesia in general. These are:

- providing a definitive airway,
- ensuring adequate oxygenation and ventilation of the lungs,
- maintaining cardiovascular stability.

A hypnotic agent is used to render the patient unconscious and analgesia given throughout the procedure to treat and prevent pain. However, the range and scale of the procedures performed during spine surgery challenge the anesthetist (and indeed the patient) sometimes more than any other subspecialty in the field of anesthesia.

This chapter will explore the approach of the anesthetist to the patient, the various pharmacological agents used and describe some of the equipment and techniques that make it possible to perform this type of surgery.

2   PREOPERATIVE ASSESSMENT

Patients presenting for spine surgery come from a broad cross section of the population. They vary in age, size, diagnosis, and comorbidity. All these will have an effect on the conduct of the anesthetic.

It is imperative that anyone having surgery is medically assessed, and this is more important as the scale of the surgery increases. Preoperative assessment clinics are a useful way of detecting morbidity either related to the presenting surgical problem or in addition to it. Usually performed a period of weeks before surgery is scheduled, medical problems can be detected and therapy optimized before the physiological insult of the surgery.

Of most relevance to anesthesia is the examination of the respiratory and cardiovascular systems. Common problems encountered are the various types of chronic obstructive airway disease:

- asthma,
- emphysema,
- chronic bronchitis.

In addition, some patients may have some form of ischemic heart disease:

- angina,
- arrhythmia,
- heart failure,
- hypertension, which will need to be controlled, as hypertension increases the risk of perioperative myocardial infarction and stroke.

2.1   SCREENING TESTS

Typical screening tests include:

- A full blood count to check for anemia and platelet problems.
- Clotting studies and serum chemistry to check renal and hepatic function.
- Blood is also checked for group and the presence of unusual antibodies that may make the provision of stored blood difficult.
- An electrocardiogram (ECG) provides a snapshot of the electrical activity of the heart. Information about rate, rhythm and blood supply to the heart is evident.
- Echocardiography is another useful test. This provides information about the structure and function of the heart. Areas of reduced movement represent damage from ischemic heart disease. The ventricles are graded for both dilatation and contraction. Importantly, the correct function and flow through the heart valves are assessed in this noninvasive test.
- A chest x-ray will be required. If there is a history of lung disease, it may be valuable to obtain pulmonary function studies, in addition to an arterial blood gas analysis with the patient breathing room air. This test requires the patient to blow into a machine and hence needs a cooperative patient. It is therefore often not possible in children. Measurements are made of the various lung volumes and these are compared to values standardized for height and sex.
- Oxygen saturation in air is a useful and easy test, though occasionally an arterial blood gas can better define a patient's respiratory disease.

2.2   AIRWAY ASSESSMENT

Airway assessment is a key skill to an anesthetist. It is performed before every anesthetic as problems of difficult intubation or ventilation can occur in any patient. In addition, patients presenting for spine surgery may have difficult airway management due to their disease process. A good example for this are patients with ankylosing spondylitis. In this disease ligamentous changes cause immobility and flexion of the spine. The patients are unable to extend their necks and often require an advanced airway technique to enable endotracheal intubation.

Instability of the cervical spine may be due to fractures, facet dislocation or ligamentous injury. Degenerative diseases such as osteoarthritis or rheumatoid arthritis can also cause instability and render the cervical spinal cord at risk. Such patients commonly have hard cervical collars or halo traction in place. Part of the purpose of these devices is to maintain cervical immobility. This can make intubation of the trachea a challenge. In these patients the safest method for establishing an airway is by awake fiberoptic intubation. In this procedure, the airway is topically anesthetized and the trachea intubated while the patient is awake with the aid of a flexible fiberoptic endoscope. Once the airway is secure and the position of the endotracheal tube checked, anesthesia is induced.

Experienced anesthetists should be able to perform or supervise the procedure with minimal discomfort to the patient. This approach is the safest as the patient is able to maintain his own airway until intubation is completed and no manipulation of the neck or head is required. If for some reason fiberoptic intubation cannot be performed, there are other, less satisfactory approaches available. In such cases, it is advantageous to discuss with the operating surgeon how much movement of the neck is allowed. Occasionally, the immobilizing device can be removed in the anesthetic room and the airway secured with a normal technique as the injury is moderately stable. In other cases, the surgeon should offer to provide in line immobilization to protect the neck, while airway manipulation proceeds and until the trachea is intubated. Prior knowledge of patients with expected difficult airway management is required so that a thorough assessment of the patient can be made, and so that the appropriate staff and equipment may be assembled.

3   CONDUCT OF ANESTHESIA

Physiological monitoring of all patients having general anesthesia is mandatory and is defined by guidelines. In the UK, the Association of Anesthetists of Great Britain and Ireland produces these guidelines.

Monitoring should begin before induction and be continued throughout the procedure and recovery period. Monitoring typically consists of:

- Continuous pulse oximetry.
- ECG.
- End tidal carbon dioxide and intermittent blood pressure readings-these are required to be recorded at regular intervals.
- Invasive monitoring of blood pressure and central venous pressure—this provides further and more immediate information about the cardiovascular condition of the patient. These monitors are particularly important for more difficult cases with greater blood loss.
- Core temperature—the esophageal route is usually used to measure the core temperature of the patient and care is taken to ensure that the patient is kept normothermic. Any fluid given to the patient is first warmed and forced warm air blowers are placed on the patient before the surgical drapes are attached. The maintenance of a normal temperature is important. Enzymes—the internal workforce of all cells in the body—are temperature sensitive and work best at normal body temperature. A fall in temperature causes a drop in efficiency and may lead to a compromised coagulation pathway (hence increased blood loss), reduced ability of the liver to metabolize drugs and reduced ability of the heart to respond to inotropes. As the core temperature falls

further the heart is more prone to arrhythmias. In addition, infection is more likely as the immune system is also compromised. In the recovery period shivering will occur; this is not only unpleasant but also dramatically increases the uptake and requirement for oxygen. In a patient with a previously compromised respiratory or cardiovascular system this may be all that is required to cause respiratory failure or myocardial infarction.

4   PHARMACOLOGICAL AGENTS

The choice of pharmacological agents used is at the discretion of the individual anesthetist. As a general principal it is more important how, rather than which particular agent is used. Induction is often accomplished with an intravenous agent, eg, propofol. However, in children and patients with challenging veins an inhalational technique may be preferable. A muscle relaxant is then used to allow intubation of the trachea and ventilation of the lungs. Maintenance of anesthesia can be achieved with any of several anesthetic vapors (commonly isoflurane or sevoflurane) or the target-controlled infusion of propofol.

There are many agents and routes to provide analgesia. The most common is the intermittent delivery of an intravenous bolus of opiate. These drugs are powerful agents with significant side effects, the most important being respiratory depression and apnea. Caution is therefore required for their safe use. Morphine is a commonly used, naturally occurring agent derived from the poppy plant. Other synthetic agents include alfentanil and fentanyl. Remifentanil is a newer agent that is finding an increasing role in spinal anesthesia. It is an ultra short-acting opiate with a half life in the plasma of only three minutes. It is therefore given by continuous intravenous infusion. Changes in infusion rate are very quickly reflected in the plasma concentration and this allows rapid changes in analgesia. This is an advantage as the stimuli that the patient is subject to during the procedure are not constant, hence the depth of anesthesia and analgesia need to be adjusted to reflect this. The anesthetist must be aware of the short duration of remifentanil when the infusion is terminated, and supplement the anesthetic with other opiates to prevent sudden acute pain from occurring. Failure to do so may make the patient uncooperative and unmanageable on emergence from anesthesia.

5   POSITIONING

Position of the patient is an important issue as most patients are prone and therefore at risk of damage to their eyes and peripheral nerves. In addition, incorrect position can lead to difficulty in ventilation and increased blood loss. The practicalities of positioning are addressed in chapter 3.3 Patient positioning for spine surgery.

6   BLOOD LOSS

The amount of blood loss during spine surgery is dependant on the operation, the number of vertebral levels operated on, and the duration of surgery. The greatest loss can be expected during deformity surgery. It can be of the order of one to two times the circulating volume of the patient. Management starts in the preoperative phase with optimization of the patient. If necessary the nutritional state of the patient may be improved by calorie and vitamin supplementation. Rarely, preoperative blood transfusion may be required to obtain an adequate hemoglobin concentration. Actual values will vary between surgical units and individual practitioners but a minimum starting hemoglobin concentration should usually be greater than 10 gdL^{-1}.

Large bore intravenous cannulae are required to keep up with ongoing blood loss. A fluid warmer is used to help prevent a fall in temperature. Heart rate, central venous pressure, urine output and blood pressure are used to guide fluid replacement. Intraoperative assessment of hemoglobin concentration and blood clotting enables the judicious use of banked blood and clotting products, eg, fresh frozen plasma and cryoprecipitate.

Red cell salvage is increasingly used in operations with associated major blood loss. This technique allows the patient's own blood to be returned to them and reduce the demand for banked blood. Close liaison with the blood bank is essential as the requirement for blood and blood products may be urgent. As greater volumes of blood are transfused there is an increased risk of compromised pulmonary function. A period of mechanical ventilation may be necessary if this is severe.

6.1   AUTOGENOUS BLOOD TRANSFUSION

Recent years have seen the demand for blood and blood products increase. This is in part due to the aging population and the greater number of operations that are performed as a result. Traditionally, there has been a great confidence in the general population regarding the quality of the blood supplied in the UK; however blood transfusion is not without risk as listed below.

Risks associated with blood transfusion are:

- ABO incompatibility,
- transmission of infection, eg, hepatitis B, hepatitis C, cytomegalovirus,
- rhesus isoimmunization,
- fluid overload,
- bacterial contamination.

Extensive screening of blood and blood donors has kept risks very small and unlike North America and most of Europe the UK has until recently continued to use blood freely. This has now changed in large part due to the appearance of new variant Creutzfeldt-Jakob disease. This is a prion disease that has now been shown to be transmissible via infected blood. As yet no tests are available to check the blood and there is a great deal of uncertainty over the size of the problem. In order to reduce risk the screening of donors has become more stringent. Most recently everyone who has received or may have received a blood transfusion in the past is now prevented from donating blood.

Thus the increasing demand for blood is being accompanied by a reducing supply. It is as a result of this that autogenous blood transfusion (red cell salvage) is becoming more popular.

6.2   THE PRACTICALITIES OF INTRAOPERATIVE RED CELL SALVAGE

Blood that is lost during the operation is collected in a reservoir. Low-pressure suction is used to minimize red cell destruction and the blood is prevented from clotting by the addition of citrate. The red cells are washed and separated by a centrifugation progress and then resuspended in 0.9% normal saline. A dedicated machine performs the process automatically and a named person who has had the appropriate training must operate it. The resulting blood has a hematocrit of 0.5–0.6 and typically one third of the blood lost is salvaged. This autogenous blood should be retransfused within six hours and should not be placed in the blood fridge during the time between collection and administration. It is worth noting that all clotting factors and platelets are lost in this process, so replacement of these may be required in the form of other blood products. This should be guided by timely tests of coagulation and a full blood count.

Simpler systems are available where blood is collected into a drain postoperatively and this is then transfused back to the patient. This is most suitable for operations where the blood loss occurs in the postoperative period, eg, in knee replacement surgery.

The advantages of red cell salvage:

- reduced requirement of banked blood,
- reduced risk of infection,
- better functioning red cells (due to normal levels of 2.3 DPG which is not present in banked blood).

Contraindications to red cell salvage:

- the presence of infection at the operative site,
- any operation for metastatic disease (cancer),
- presence of iodine or iodine-containing products in the wound.

7   MONITORING OF SPINAL CORD FUNCTION

Spinal cord function can be monitored intraoperatively using several types of evoked potential. Stimuli may be applied peripherally and measured centrally (somatosensory-evoked potentials, or SSEPs) or vice versa (motor-evoked potentials, or MEPs). The amplitude of signals that cross the area of the operation are measured; a drop of 50% from baseline would be significant.

Spinal cord function may be altered by hypotension, hypoxia, or surgical misadventure. The anesthetic agents are chosen to avoid interaction with evoked potential monitoring. This subject is more widely addressed in chapter 1.3 Spinal cord monitoring.

8   POSTOPERATIVE CARE

Attention to detail is the key to effective postoperative care. Of primary concern is ensuring that appropriately trained staff, in the appropriate setting, care for the appropriate patient. Many complications can be prevented or their severity reduced if detected early. Accurate, regular recording of vital signs will highlight a patient that is not progressing as planned and appropriate action can then be taken.

Routine observations consist of:

- oxygen saturation,
- respiratory rate,
- heart rate,
- urine output,
- blood pressure,
- temperature,
- full blood count and serum chemistry to guide intravenous therapy, and
- frequent neurological assessment is important to detect potentially treatable nerve or spinal cord compression.

Analgesic choices usually consist of morphine via a patient-controlled analgesia device in addition to simple oral analgesics. Paracetamol and nonsteroidal anti-inflammatory agents are commonly used. Other options include epidural or paravertebral infusions of opiates and/or local anesthetics.

9 SPECIAL CONSIDERATIONS FOR CERVICAL SURGERY

Special preparations should be taken when extubating the trachea of a patient who has undergone anterior and/or posterior cervical spine surgery. These patients are at particular risk of airway complications. Retraction and distortion of the trachea is necessary surgically to expose the cervical spine. This, in combination with the presence of an endotracheal tube, may result in airway edema, which in turn may cause total airway obstruction when the endotracheal tube is removed. Bleeding into the soft tissues of the neck postoperatively may also cause distortion or obstruction of the airway. Some patients undergoing cervical spine surgery will be placed in a cervical collar or halo jacket prior to emergence from anesthesia. In this case emergency reintubation of the trachea if needed is difficult or impossible. Therefore, before extubation of the trachea, it is advisable to deflate the balloon on the endotracheal tube, occlude the endotracheal tube, and determine whether the patient is able to breathe around the tube. If not, the patient may need a period of postoperative ventilation to allow the edema to resolve. Another option is to insert an airway exchange catheter through the endotracheal tube before its removal. That way, if the patient needs emergency reintubation, the airway exchange catheter will serve as a conduit to reestablish tracheal intubation quickly.

10 ANESTHESIA FOR THORACOTOMY

Operations on the anterior part of the spine above the diaphragm require an incision to be made in the chest wall. It is possible to ventilate only one lung and let the other deflate. This provides easier surgical access to the spine. There are various methods to accomplish this.

In adults and patients down to about 30 kg, double lumen tubes can selectively ventilate the lungs (**Fig 3.2-1a–b**).

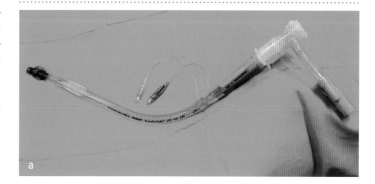

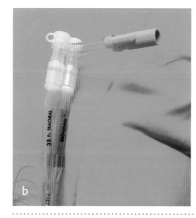

Fig 3.2-1a–b
a Double lumen endotracheal tube.
b Double lumen endotracheal tube—detail of connection to breathing circuit.
(Reproduced with kind permission of Cook Medical.)

An alternative is the use of a balloon-tipped catheter (bronchial blocker). This device is passed under direct vision with the aid of a fiberoptic scope and placed in the main bronchus of the lung to be deflated. Once inflated, the balloon prevents gas flow to the selected lung, which deflates as the gas within it is absorbed (**Fig 3.2-2a–d**).

In pediatric patients it is often not possible to isolate the lungs as the bronchial tree is so small. Instead the lung is gently held away by appropriate retractors.

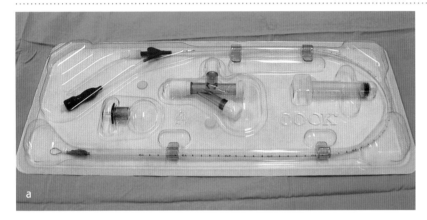
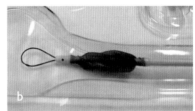
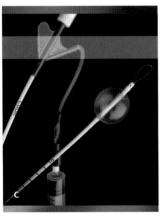
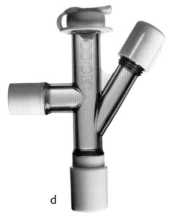

Fig 3.2-2a–d
a   Bronchial blocker set in packaging.
b   Bronchial blocker—detail of tip.
c   Balloon inflated.
d   Detail of circuit connector.
(Reproduced with kind permission of Cook Medical.)

Adequate oxygenation and ventilation during one lung ventilation is often a challenge and successful management requires significant experience.

Pain following a thoracotomy is intense and requires significant attention. The options include all those previously mentioned; however, the best analgesia is a mixture of local anesthetic and an opiate, provided by epidural or paravertebral infusion.

The provision of anesthesia for spine surgery may be challenging. Success relies on the anticipation of events intraoperatively and anticipation of complications postoperatively. Adequate preparation and assessment of the patient is paramount. Massive blood loss is common and should be expected.

11   SUGGESTION FOR FURTHER READING

Raw DA, Beattie JK, Hunter JM (2003) Anaesthesia for spinal surgery in adults. *Br J Anaesth;* 91(6):886–904.

3.3   PATIENT POSITIONING FOR SPINE SURGERY

1   INTRODUCTION

Spine surgery addresses the full extent of the spinal column from the occipital to the coccygeal region. Surgical approaches may be made from the anterior, lateral, and posterior aspects. Appropriate positioning of the patient is essential to allow the surgical procedure to be performed correctly. Insufficient care in transferring and positioning the patient can have a damaging effect on many body systems. The respiratory, cardiovascular, and nervous systems can all be affected. Complications may occur, which involves damage to skin, muscle, and other soft tissues. Injuries such as joint dislocation or, in extreme cases, pathological fracture, may occur. Such instances can never be justified.

Individually, therefore, each operating room personnel (ORP) must fully understand the factors that affect positioning, during the preoperative, anesthetic, and postoperative phases of care [1], as well as the associated hazards.

The primary goal is threefold to ensure the safe transfer of the patient from the trolley/bed to the operating table, achieving safe and secure positioning for the duration of the surgery, and finally, safely transferring the patient from the operating table back to the trolley/bed.

Although the final responsibility for the safety and efficacy of patient positioning rests with the surgeon in partnership with the anesthetist, successful patient positioning can only be achieved by the cooperation, coordination, and full attention of the multidisciplinary operating room (OR) team.

It is of paramount importance to remember that during surgery the anesthetized patient is entirely defenseless, unable to communicate, and deprived of both voluntary and involuntary protective responses. While in the OR the health and safety of the patient is, quite literally, in the hands of the OR team.

2   AIMS

The aims of the patient positioning are:

- to provide a comfortable and safe position for the patient during surgery,
- to allow the surgeon good surgical access to the spine,
- to allow the anesthetist to access the airway and peripheral lines at all times,
- to allow access of additional equipment, eg, microscope, x-ray, C-arm/portable machine, and spinal cord monitoring,
- to achieve all of the above without detriment to the patient's well being.

3   GENERAL REFLECTION

3.1   PLANNING

"Proper planning prevents predictably poor performance."

Before the patient enters the OR the following is to consider:

- Is the correct operating table in the OR?
  Depending on the surgery and type of operating tables available, it may be necessary to change tables to achieve the required patient position. The patient's weight may also be a consideration as large patients may require a heavy table. A radiolucent table top may be required for x-ray screening of the spine.
- Is the operating table in good working order?
  A defective operating table is hazardous.
- Is the operating table positioned appropriately?
  Relocating an operating table after the patient has been transferred is a dangerous maneuver for both the patient and the team.
- Are all the necessary table attachments and props available and in good working order?
  Unavailable or defective equipment builds in delay and hazards.
- Alternative attachments/props and padding may be required, what is the availability?
  Patients are individuals and are not identical, therefore alternative options could become a major advantage.
- Are sufficient personnel available to undertake the transfer?
  Attempting to position a patient for surgery without adequate assistance puts both the patient and staff at risk of injury; the required number of personnel for transfer is six team members.

---

4   GENERAL HAZARD

4.1   TRAUMATIC INJURIES

During any transfer maneuver, the head must be supported and can only be moved in such a way that the anatomical alignment of the cervical spine is maintained throughout. The extremities, particularly hands and fingers, can be inadvertently trapped prior to transfer. Injury occurs when this goes unnoticed and an attempt is made to lift or turn the patient without ensuring that they are free to move. Checking is essential prior to transfer to ensure that the limbs are free from obstruction to movement.

All anesthetic, intravenous, and drainage tubing is hazardous, as is any attached monitoring equipment. The equipment must be either able to move with the patient, or the leads/tubing must be of sufficient length not to impede movement. In some instances, it may be advantageous to temporarily disconnect monitors or tubing (clamping or cap as appropriate) prior to transfer and reconnect them after positioning has been completed. Where leads/tubing are left attached during transfer, check that their movement is unobstructed and that they will not become trapped underneath the patient following transfer. Limb injury can also occur if they are allowed to trail or flail during the transfer process. It is important to ensure that the arms and legs are secured and moved in concert with the patient's body. Shearing or tearing of the underlying tissues can occur when the patient's skin is taut during transfer, so the patient must never be dragged across the two points of transfer.

4.2   POSITION-RELATED INJURIES

Care must be taken to avoid position-related injuries both in the process of transferring/positioning, and in the final position itself. Unnatural movement of the torso, head, or limbs, hyperextension, and extremes of final positioning can all lead to serious injury, potentially damaging soft tissue, joints, or nerves. Some complex procedures require changing the position of the patient intraoperatively. Where this is intended, additional consideration must be given to how that maneuver is to be achieved. Will changing the position itself give rise to positioning injuries, hyperextension, etc? Are limbs or areas of soft tissue in danger of being trapped by the change of position? Will tube or monitoring cables be pulled out of position or become disconnected?

4.3   PRESSURE-RELATED INJURIES

Once positioned, the patient will remain motionless for the duration of the operation, which in spine surgery can be several hours. This is an unnatural situation and the soft tissues are vulnerable to damage caused simply by prolonged pressure. Pressure sores and nerve injury can occur as a result. Bony prominences and superficially placed nerve structures are particularly at risk. Careful positioning and the use of padding and limb supports must be employed to eliminate or at least dissipate these pressure effects and avoid necrosis which is a potentially traumatic complication. All soft tissues are at risk during transfers and surgery. Pressure sores can occur if the surgery transmits in excess of 2 hours of static pressure, and excessive pressure is placed on blood vessels [1]. This leads to vascular compromise, creating the following complications:

- deficiency in oxygen,
- compromise of nutrition,
- development of metabolic waste [2].

Extra precautions must be given to the breasts and male genitals when in the prone position, ensuring no unnecessary pressure or friction has been applied to them.

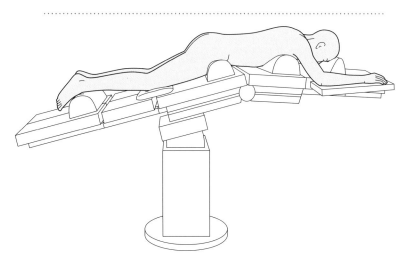

Fig 3.3-1
A patient in the prone position.

5   COMMON SURGICAL POSITIONS

Depending on the operative approach and which level of the spine is being addressed, the required patient position will be:

- prone,
- supine,
- lateral, or
- knee-chest.

Once the patient has been anesthetized and all other required procedures have been performed, eg, central lines, long lines, and urinary catheterization. The patient may also require cervical traction (see chapter 3.4 Spinal traction). The team should conduct the transfer in a coordinated manner onto the operating table.

It is important to identify a coordinator for the transfer. Generally, the anesthetist will take on this role; they are controlling the patient's head and airway. (The only exception the author has identified is with cervical surgery. Due to the possible instability of the cervical spine, the surgeon may wish to be in control of the transfer).

5.1   PRONE POSITION

The prone position (**Fig 3.3-1**) allows surgical access to the posterior elements of the whole spinal column, from the occipital to the coccygeal region.

The majority of spine surgery is performed with the patient in the prone position. Unfortunately, at the present time this means that some manual handling is inevitable. Extra care must be taken to protect the team's own backs during the transfer of the patient.

Craig [3] describes a method of turning the patient into the prone position using bed sheets. This technique may be ideal in a general specialty but due to the length of spine surgery can add a potential risk to the patient. Putting linen between jelly pressure pads and the patient poses a risk to patients with poor skin condition, as sheets are coarse in texture and have a tendency to wrinkle under patients no matter what position they are in. Further, if pulled they can cause shearing or tearing of the epidermis.

Positioning aids
The aids required will generally be dependant on the operating table used in the OR, the preference of the surgeon, and to some extent the weight and size of the patient.

The most commonly used props for this position are:

- Montreal mattress rolls, or wedge and bolster in which to accommodate the patient's torso, allowing the abdomen to be free of pressure.
- Arm supports, as the arms will be placed alongside the head where possible. A variation on this is surgery on the posterior elements of the cervical spine; the patient's arms should be placed alongside the torso.
- Head rings, horseshoe, pads, or pillows are used to accommodate the head. This should be placed in the most natural position possible without causing airway obstruction or putting unnecessary pressure on the patient's chin. Usually the patient's head is placed to the side.
- Pillows, jelly pads, or padding should be used under the knees and feet; the feet require slight elevation to protect the plantar nerves.

5.2   SUPINE POSITION

The supine position (**Fig 3.3-2**) is universal to all patients from the time of their arrival in the department until they are positioned for surgery, the administration of anesthetic and subsequent transfer.

The supine position allows surgical access to the anterior body of the cervical and lumbar column. In extreme cases of deformity or high thoracic fractures and diseases, a sternal split would be performed in this position.

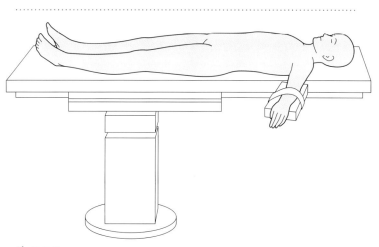

Fig 3.3-2
A patient in the supine position.

Positioning aids
The most commonly used aids for this position are:

- Jelly pads the full length of the operating table to protect the bony prominences and skin from the neck to the patient's ankles.
- Pillows, cervical beanbag, or horseshoe to accommodate the head.
- Heel pads to raise the ankles slightly.
- Arm supports—IV access is routinely required, so arms are placed on arm boards in the crucifix position, being careful not to overextend the arms, as this can lead to nerve damage.

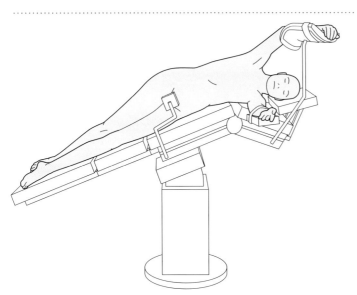

Fig 3.3-3
A patient in the lateral position.

5.3   LATERAL POSITION

The lateral position (**Fig 3.3-3**) allows surgical access to the anterior thoracic and thorocolumbar column. In cases of deformity or disease, this position also allows access for anterior and posterior in a combined situation.

This position requires extra care during the turn and must be conducted with an adequate number of team members. Care must be taken to ensure all pressure points are addressed correctly.

Positioning aids
The most commonly used aids for this position are:

- Vacuum beanbag, which cushions support and lifts the torso from the operating table.
- Pillows or jelly head ring to place the patient's head in as normal a position as possible.
- Pillows or pads placed between the legs to protect the bony prominences.
- Heel pads, jelly pads, or pillows placed under heels to raise them from the operating table.
- The dependent arm is bent at the elbow and laid alongside the head and shoulders.
- The upper arm placed on a ball and socket armrest with jelly pads or padding to allow the arm to be placed in a natural position.
- Straps and abdominal prop to stabilize and secure the patient to the operating table.

5.4   KNEE-CHEST POSITION

The knee-chest position (**Fig 3.3-4**) allows surgical access to the lumbar posterior elements and segments. The advantage of this position is that it opens up the facet joints.

This position may offer superior access for the surgeon, but at a cost of extra maneuvering for the team. Due to their anesthetic state, patients are at their most vulnerable when being turned into this position. The type of operating table used will determine how much manual handling the team must undertake to achieve this position.

Positioning aids
The most commonly used aids for this position are:

- Knee-chest prop to support the patient's buttocks.
- Roll or prop placed under the chest once the turn has been made.
- Jelly pads, pillows, or pads placed on the knee-chest table attachment to cushion the knees.
- Jelly head ring or pillows to accommodate the head.
- Arm boards with jelly pads placed to allow the arms to be extended alongside the head.

Both operating tables and positioning props may vary according to the surgeon's preference and the environment in the OR.

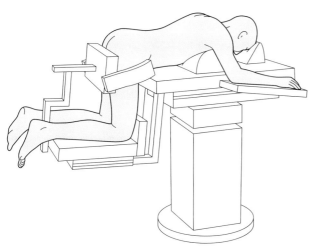

Fig 3.3-4
A patient in the knee-chest position.

6   COMPLICATIONS AND RISKS

Restricted respiration
In the prone and knee-chest position the diaphragm compresses against the abdominal wall leading to poor expansion of the lungs. The use of the Montreal mattress/rolls or wedge-shaped props allows the abdomen to fall into the gap created, thus allowing the diaphragm to move freely and the lungs to expand.

In the lateral position pressure and tension on the upper intercostals and lumbar muscles may interfere with the breathing. During thoracic spine surgery the patient is ventilated on one lung, and may even require disruption or division of the diaphragm. This is a requirement in which the surgeon gains access to the upper levels of the thoracic anterior body of the spine.

Diminished and/or compromised venous return
Pressure in the inferior vena cava from the abdominal contents and wall can lead to venous engorgement of the torso and spine. This increases the blood volume at the operative site, and is a major positioning complication when the patient is prone, knee-chest, or lateral. Large and obese patients are particularly susceptible to this complication.

There is also a risk of thrombosis; antiembolism stockings or an electric deep vein thrombosis prophylaxis system should be used to reduce the risk.

Neural damage
The nerves are susceptible to stretching and damage, both in relation to transfer, lengthy procedures and poor positioning. This can lead to a temporary, long-term or permanent damage. The injury is caused by ischemia, compression, traction, or laceration.

Highlighted are those nerves at risk with regard to spine surgery.

- Radius and ulna—poor arm board positioning in the supine position can damage these nerves, thus the arms should not be extended more than 90°. When in the lateral position extra care should be taken to prevent the lower arm becoming trapped by the torso.
- Brachial plexus—when the head is suddenly twisted away from the abducted shoulders, or the head is not supported in the lateral position.
- Plantar nerves—when the feet and calves are not raised slightly away from the table.
- Perineal nerves—when the lateral aspects of the lower knee are not protected with pillows and padding.

Eye injury
When the patient is in the prone position for any length of time the eyes are at risk from corneal abrasions and conjunctive edema. In extreme conditions this can lead to blindness. The eyes must be well padded and taped prior to turning in the prone or knee-chest position. During spine surgery this is routine for all positions. This is to both protect the eyes and securely maintain the endotracheal tube during surgery.

Bony prominences

The common sites for vascular compromise over bony prominences during surgery are the scapulae, elbows, sacrum, heels, and the greater trochanter [4]. All can be at risk during supine and lateral spine surgery.

The forehead, nose, iliac crest, and knees are other bony areas where vascular compromise may develop during surgery in the prone and knee-chest positions. These may lead to pressure sores if not adequately padded and supported. Thus, the need for pressure relief for all bony prominences is of paramount importance.

It is vitally important that all the risk areas are checked following the final positioning, prior to the skin preparation and surgical drapes being applied. This must be seen as a team effort undertaken by all ORP and other medical staff. Postoperative pain from positioning is common, and the lengthy duration of many spine surgery procedures increases this possibility.

7   ASSOCIATED RISKS

Hypothermia

The patient should remain covered as long as possible in order to preserve dignity. This also minimizes heat loss. Warming blankets are a great asset in maintaining body heat, helping to lessen the risk of hypothermia due to the extensive surgical time. Hypothermia can contribute to an increase in surgical bleeding, postoperative discomfort, and impaired wound healing. The patients most at risk are children, the elderly, and the physically slight of build. Tudor [5] looked at patients' temperatures in relation to loss of body heat during the preoperative period. By a scientific approach he dentified nine risk factors thus allowing the ORP to predict which patients were at risk and the level of intervention required to address the loss in body temperature. This study is recommended for further reading to explain the importance of maintaining body heat pre- and postoperatively.

Log rolling

A log roll is a patient-handling maneuver designed to minimize movement of the structures of the spine while turning the patient. It is used with patients who may be at risk of developing neurological deficits as a result of structural instability of the spinal tissues. During log rolling the patient is moved in a coordinated manner that maintains spinal alignment at all times.

If there is any uncertainty as to the stability of the patient's spine, or in the instance of multiple system trauma, the patients must always be log rolled.

In an ideal world, a team of eight is required to achieve the transfer with total safety in the OR. However, due to staffing levels within departments, this procedure may have to be performed with six team members. As with all lifts the coordinator is in control of the move.

The team should be placed alongside the patient and at the receiving side of the operating table in order of height, the tallest being at the patient's shoulders and the smallest at the feet.

The role of the coordinator is to:

- Ensure the operating table, trolley, or bed is the correct height for the move.
- Ensure the team involved in the move is comfortable and ready to start.
- Ensure the team is aware of the signal to start (generally this is a count of 3).
- Give clear instructions to the team during the move.
- Reassess spinal alignment once the patient is positioned.

The role of the team is:

- Coordinator supports the head and neck.
- Team member 1 supports the shoulders and the spine as far as the rib cage.
- Team member 2 supports the ribcage to the pelvis.
- Team member 3 supports the pelvis and legs—this team member's hand should touch or overlap with member 2 to facilitate coordination of movement and to maximize support to the patient's spine.
- Team member 4 supports the feet and catheter tube and bag if in situ.
- Team member 5 will mirror 3 on receiving the patient.
- Team member 6 will mirror 2 on receiving the patient.
- Team member 7 will mirror 1 on receiving the patient.

If only six team members are available the move is still possible but could potentially put the patient at risk.

In order to prevent any untoward incidents, team members must be clear about their role, and hospitals should have specific guidelines for log rolling in place in order to clarify these roles and responsibilities.

All team members associated with the operating department, whatever their level, have a role to play in patient safety. Patients that come to our department are vulnerable, whether in a conscious or unconscious state, and have a right to be kept safe. It is the responsibility of the ORP to protect and preserve their safety and dignity. This applies from the time they arrive in the department, to the time they return to the ward.

8   BIBLIOGRAPHY

1. **Clarke P, Jones J** (1998) Brigden's Operating Department Practice. Edinburgh: Churchill Livingstone.
2. **Taylor M, Campbell C** (1999) Back to basics–Patient care in the operating department (1). *Br J of Theatre Nurs;* 9(6):272–275.
3. **Craig K** (2003) Prone positioning made easy. *Br J Perioper Nurs;* 13(12):522–527.
4. **Hartley L** (2003) Reducing pressure damage in the operating theatre. *Br J Perioper Nurs;* 13(6):249–254.
5. **Tudor M** (1994) Scaling the patient's temperature–Part 1. *Br J Theatre Nurs;* 3(11):20–23.

3　OPERATIVE KNOWLEDGE FOR SPINE SURGERY

3.4　SPINAL TRACTION

3.4   SPINAL TRACTION

1   INDICATIONS

Spinal traction can be used for many different applications.

Indications include:

- Reduction of spinal fractures and dislocations. Most commonly used in cervical spine facet joint dislocations.
- To temporarily maintain normal or acceptable spinal alignment in order to prevent neurological deterioration. This can be posttrauma or after stage one of two-stage operations.
- In the treatment of spinal fractures. It can be used to hold fractures in an acceptable position until healed or stable enough to be managed in a collar.
- To improve spinal deformity. For example it can be used to slowly correct scoliosis or spondylolisthesis after osteotomy/release.
- To hold a position of the head and neck during spine surgery, eg, some surgeons use Gardner-Wells tongs to hold position during anterior cervical discectomy.

2   COMMON METHODS EMPLOYED

The most common method is occipitocervical traction. The concept of this dates back to Hippocrates and Galen. It has been widely used since the development of Crutchfield tongs in 1933. Currently, the two commonest methods used are Gardner-Wells tongs and halo traction. For cervical traction 4.5 kg (10 lbs) is generally regarded as a reasonable weight to hold a position. If planning to reduce a dislocation, 4.5 kg (10 lbs) are first attached then an x-ray is taken. A further 2.3 kg (5 lbs) is then added, with a new x-ray sequentially until reduction is achieved. It is estimated that 4.5 kg (10 lbs) plus 2.3 kg (5 lbs) for each additional level of injury will be required. If no reduction has occurred by 22.7 kg (50 lbs), most surgeons will proceed to open reduction. However, there is no recognized upper limit for traction and some authors have suggested up to 63.6 kg (140 lbs) is safe.

2.1   GARDNER-WELLS TONGS

Developed in the 1980s, these are a safe, simple reliable piece of equipment (**Fig 3.4-1a–b**).

The pins are inserted just above the ear below the maximum diameter of the skull. The AP position of the pins can be adjusted by small amounts to gain increased flexion or extension during traction. The skin is prepared with iodine or chlorhexidine prior to pin insertion. The pins are spring loaded and it is accepted that a 1–2 mm protrusion of the pins is a safe distance of insertion. This is equivalent to three finger tightness (the tightness obtained by using the tumb, index, and middle finger). Weights can then be attached via traction apparatus.

2.2   MAYFIELD OR DORO HEAD CLAMP

This equipment is very useful for holding an exact head/neck position (**Fig 3.4-2a–b**). It is commonly used for cervical spine posterior surgery and occipitocervical fusions. The exact flexion, extension, and rotation can be accurately held to maintain reduction. Stability gained by using this equipment allows safe use of drills and other instruments without fear of the spine moving. It attaches to the operating table as an extension and contains a main C piece and three sterile pins. It is important to check the apparatus is securely attached to the table prior to pin insertion.

The head position is held by one surgeon, being careful to keep hands clear of the pin insertion area. There are two pins on one side and a single pin on the other. The clamp is then squeezed onto the skull by a second surgeon. The screw is then

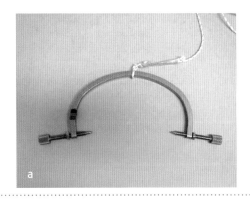
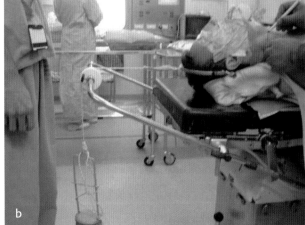

Fig 3.4-1a–b
a Gardner-Wells tongs.
b In situ with weights
   applied.

tightened to 60 lbs (27.2 kg) or three threads showing for adults. Smaller pins, clamps, and different pressures are used for pediatric patients as set out by product manufacturers' guidelines.

2.3   HALO TRACTION

Halo traction is the other commonly used traction system (**Fig 3.4-3a–b**). This uses four points of attachment to the skull, compared with two in Gardner-Wells. This is therefore a more stable construct. Using torque screws may also be safer than a spring-loaded mechanism. The disadvantage of this system is that the anterior pin sites can leave a visible scar in an important cosmetic site.

Halo traction is especially useful if the traction is likely to be changed to definitive treatment with a halo jacket. For details of insertion see 2.4 Halo jacket, in this chapter.

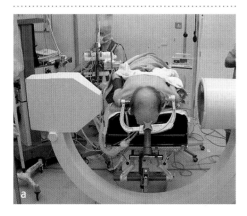

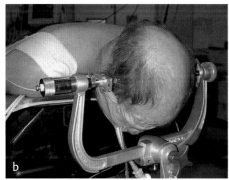

Fig 3.4-2a–b
Doro head clamp in situ.

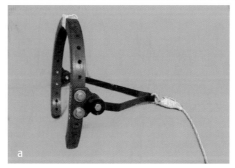

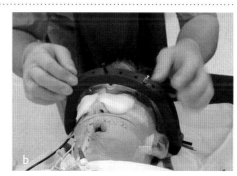

Fig 3.4-3a–b
a Carbon fiber halo.
b Halo being applied in preparation for halo jacket.

2.4   HALO JACKET

First used by Perry and Nickels in 1959 for cervical spine fusion in poliomyelitis patients. The halo is made of carbon fiber or titanium so making it MRI compatible. The jacket can be made of plaster of paris but preformed plastic is more commonly used. This technique provides the best orthotic immobilization for upper and lower cervical spine fractures. It is less effective in the mid cervical spine.

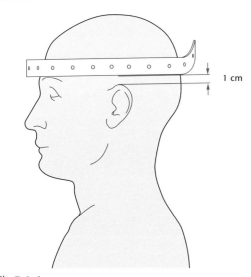

Fig 3.4-4
Halo position.

Traction is provided between the jacket and the halo ring. It cannot provide traction as powerful as tongs/halo traction. It is not effective as the only form of stabilization in, for example, a patient following a vertebrectomy. Gravity overcomes the halo traction and kyphosis may occur. If a cage or bone strut is present then the halo would be sufficient. Common uses are for the treatment of atlas and axis fractures, and to hold pediatric patients postlaminectomy for intradural tumor. It can also be used for the treatment of cervical facet dislocations [1].

Halo ring application
Halos come in varying sizes and it is important to measure the patient prior to the procedure. The head circumference is measured directly or templates are used to estimate the correct halo ring size.

The ring should allow 1–2 cm clearance from the skull. The halo should be positioned 1 cm above the eyebrow anteriorly and 1 cm above the ears posteriorly in the occipitoparietal area (**Fig 3.4-4**). It is essential that the halo be sufficiently far down onto the supraorbital ridge to get a satisfactory grip in the outer table, especially if the frontal bones are sloping. It is also important to make sure the halo is below the maximum skull diameter posteriorly to avoid slippage.

The halo is applied around the skull in the required position and temporarily held with three positioning pins with plastic pads (**Fig 3.4-5**). The patient must shut their eyes prior to pin insertion.

The pin sites are now selected and cleaned with betadine or chlorhexidene. The skin and periosteum are infiltrated with local anesthetic. Anteriorly, the pins should be in the outer 1/3 of the eyebrow to avoid supraorbital nerve injury. The pins posteriorly need to avoid the temporal bone as it can be very thin. The pins are hand tightened down to the skin. The skin can either be incised or the pin can be allowed to penetrate the skin itself. As the pins penetrate the skin they will gain purchase in the outer table of the skull (**Fig 3.4-6**).

Opposing pins are tightened sequentially by hand and finally with the torque screwdriver up to a maximum of 0.28 kg/cm^2 for children and up to 0.56 kg/cm^2 for adults. Tightening over 0.56 kg/cm^2 has been shown not to significantly increase the stability and will increase the risk of inner table perforation. Care is required in an elderly patient that over tightening is not performed as this can cause inner table penetration. Once the pins are applied, the temporary positioning pins can be removed.

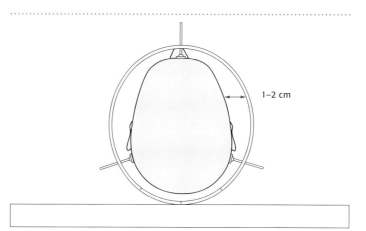

Fig 3.4-5
Halo held with temporary pins.

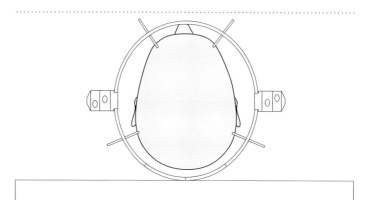

Fig 3.4-6
Halo and pins in position.

The jacket again has to be sized prior to the procedure. A circumferential measurement is taken at the nipple level and the appropriate size selected. The jacket is then attached as per manufacturers' instructions. A better construct is achieved if the rods are symmetrical and parallel (**Fig 3.4-7a–b**).

X-rays are performed and the position of the spine is checked. Adjustments are made as necessary.

The pins need to be retorqued at 24 hours, then at 3 days, and thereafter weekly until the halo is removed.

The pin sites need to be cleaned with betadine every day. The pins should be replaced if there is significant loosening or infection.

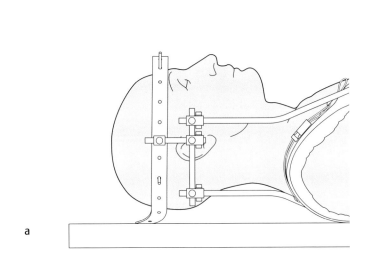

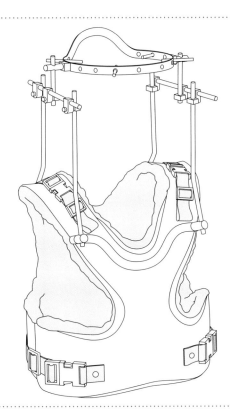

a

b

Fig 3.4-7a–b
a Halo with jacket rods.
b Halo jacket.

3   COMPLICATIONS

The complications of traction and halo jacket immobilization are common but the majority are minor (**Table 3.4-1**) [2].

Pin site loosening is treated by pin replacement. Pin site infections are usually well controlled with a short course of appropriate antibiotics. Other complications can be kept to a minimum by strict and meticulous technique.

Complication	%
Pin loosening	36
Pin infection	20
Pin site pain	18
Pressure sores	11
Visible cosmetic scars	9
Neurological injury	2
Dysphagia	2
Pin site hemorrhage	1
Dural puncture	1
Intercranial abscess	Less than 1

Table 3.4-1
Complications of traction and halo jacket immobilization.

4   BIBLIOGRAPHY

1. **Beyer CA, Cabanela ME, Berquist TH** (1991) Unilateral facet dislocations and fracture-dislocations of the cervical spine. *J Bone Joint Surg Br;* 73(6):977–981.
2. **Garfin SR** (1989) *Complications of Spine Surgery (Management of Complications in Orthopedics)*. Baltimore: Williams & Wilkins.

3.5   UNIVERSAL INSTRUMENTS USED FOR SPINE SURGERY

1   INTRODUCTION

Instruments play a key part in any surgical procedure. They vary both in structure and design, depending on the role they have to perform. Surgeons have individual preferences, but they will accept universal trays for exposure, prevalent spine surgery, and closure of spinal procedures. It is the responsibility of operating room personnel (ORP) to have knowledge of each individual instrument's role, care, maintenance, and decontamination process.

High standards and strict compliance with the decontamination process is extremely important when dealing with surgical instruments. The increase in infection rates of variant Creutzfeldt-Jakob disease (CJD), hospital-acquired infection, and antibiotic resistant bacteria are major issues within healthcare today. Due to the highly publicized nature of these diseases, particularly CJD, there is now greater general public awareness of these issues, and subsequently a heightened anxiety on the part of all ORP to ensure that infection control issues are being appropriately addressed.

2   INSTRUMENTS

Most surgical instruments are produced from a high grade of stainless steel. Flexibility and pliability is dependent on individual instruments and their usage.

Stainless steel contains the following elements and is classified by the amount of [1]:

- iron,
- carbon,
- chromium.

The handling of instruments is a very important part of the scrub role. They should be passed in a decisive manner; the handle should be placed directly and firmly in the surgeon's hand. The working end of the instrument should not be handled by any scrub member of the team, as this will be directly inserted into the cavity, tissues, and bone. To prevent injury to both the patient and scrub team members, blades must always be presented inside a receiver.

All trays required for the procedure must be checked at the outset to ensure they are conforming (complete as per tray list); nonconforming trays may delay the procedure or may lead to the surgery being abandoned. Preparation of trolleys should only commence immediately before the start of the procedure, as this will help to safeguard against contamination.

To avoid damage to any instrument it should only be used for the purpose for which it was designed. If instrumentation is abused or misused, it becomes blunt or possibly misshapen, which may prove to be unsafe in some circumstances.

General spinal trays should contain the following instruments:

- Blade handle to mount both large and small blades.
- Scissors for cutting both tissue and sutures.
- Holding forceps for tissues, artery/vein, dissecting, swabs, and needles.
- Retractors—both self retaining and hand held for tissue and nerve root retraction.
- Accessories—suction ends of at least three different diameters, dissecting probes, bipolar and diathermy forceps, metal ruler, sharp and blunt hooks (**Fig 3.5-1a**).

In addition to general instruments the spine surgeon will require orthopedic instrumentation such as:

- Osteotomes of various size cutting edges, hammer, three sizes of gouges.
- Bone curettes, nibblers, punch, rongeurs, and cutters.
- Soft-tissue rongeurs.
- Cobbs elevators of varying sizes (**Fig 3.5-1b**).

To apply any form of implant to the bone the scrub ORP should have the specialized instruments and implant trays available from the preferred company at the start of the surgery.

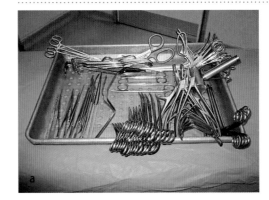

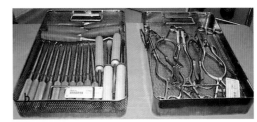

Fig 3.5-1a–b
General spinal and orthopedic instruments.

3   PROCESSING OF INSTRUMENTS

Line [2] states: "Decontamination covers all aspects of reprocessing of reusable equipment." Strict control of sterilizing instruments is bound by the Consumer Protection Act of 1987 and each company's product liability. It is vital that each instrument has been through a recordable traceability system within each unit, so the tracking system may be audited; this allows all instruments to be traced to a particular patient [3]. Decontamination is achieved through a strict process, and each instrument must go through the appropriate process to achieve the optimum level of sterility (**Fig 3.5-2**).

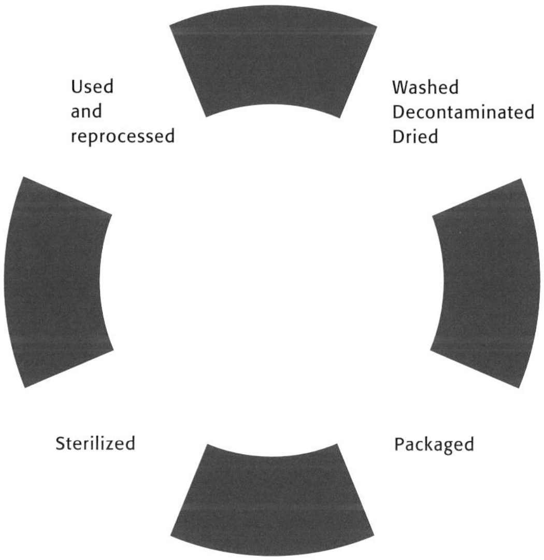

Miller [4] classifies the outcomes under three headings:

- Cleansing—removal of blood, bodily fluids, and soil.
- Disinfecting—removal of many or all microorganisms, apart from highly resistant bacterial endospores, through the use of liquid chemicals or wet pasteurization.
- Sterilization—complete removal or obliteration of microbial life through:
  – steam (under pressure),
  – ethylene oxide gas,
  – dry heat,
  – gas plasma,
  – liquid chemicals.

Sterilization is defined by Hewitson [5] as a "process used to render an object free from all viable microorganisms, but absolute sterility is unattainable". All instruments should be cleaned as soon as possible after use, checked for damage and only be returned to the trays if in good working order. They must only be used in a sterile condition; if the team is not confident the instrument is sterile it must be returned for reprocessing.

Used
and
reprocessed

Washed
Decontaminated
Dried

Sterilized

Packaged

Fig 3.5-2
The cycle of reprocessing instruments.

3.1   WASHING, DRYING, AND LUBRICATING

Washing can be achieved in three different ways, hand, machine, or ultrasonic. Most instruments can be machine washed, allowing the tracking process to be activated from the start of the procedure. Drying is completed via the machine cycle and then followed by lubrication.

Hand washing must only be attempted under strict conditions:

- Staff—must use appropriate clothing to protect against sharps injury, splashing, and aerosols.
- Cool or warm water only to be used.
- A neutral pH detergent must be used.
- Nonabrasive cleaning solutions.
- Lumina instruments must be flushed through with cold water.
- All instruments must have a final rinse with pure filtered water.
- All instruments must be dried thoroughly to prevent corrosion at instrument joints.

Machine washing is by far the best method for instruments if the item allows. It removes up to 60% of blood and protein deposits depending on the pH efficiency of the detergent used [1]. This process also decreases the risks highlighted above to the staff in the sterilization department, and has the advantage of a drying cycle.

Ultrasonic cleaners produce high-frequency sound waves which are converted into mechanical vibrations, causing microscopic bubbles to form. This is a highly effective form of drawing out tissue deposits, as up to 90% of this matter can be removed using this process [1].

Lubrication

Manufacturers of all instruments recommend lubrication before sterilization, particularly when ultrasonic cleaning has been used, as this process removes all traces of previous lubricant applications. Lubricants contain antibacterial and rust-inhibiting agents, but still allow steam to penetrate during the autoclaving stage to prevent the formation of bacteria.

Packaging

This part of the process can vary in each hospital due to the large amount of packaging material and trays/tins available for purchase. Nevertheless, all instruments must be appropriately contained or wrapped prior to the autoclave process. At this stage, the mechanism in place to identify sterility of the instruments after the autoclave process is applied, eg, autoclave tape, which is pink in color until sterilization, when it turns brown. This is then accepted as sterilized and ready for use. All singly packed items must be double wrapped and checked prior to use for damaged packaging. All trays/tins or singly wrapped instruments must have a clear label with preferred tracking method used. If perforation, missed sealant edges, tears, or tins with absent filters are found, the instruments must be discarded and returned to the sterilizing area.

Autoclaving—steam heat

These machines play a major role in the OR setting, and are used to sterilize the majority of instruments today. There are two common autoclave temperature cycles:

- 134°–137°C which sterilizes in approximately 3 minutes. Including the drying time the whole cycle takes 30 minutes
- 121°–124°C which sterilizes in approximately 15 minutes.

Ethylene oxide

Ethylene oxide is used when the instrument or surgical equipment is sensitive to the rigors of the steam cycle. The problem with this procedure is that the instruments are sent away to an external specialist company for processing, therefore resources must be examined carefully to cope with the processing and return of equipment, ie, either extra sterile instrumentation should be available or services designed around the estimated time of process.

Disinfectants

There are two liquid disinfecting solutions used in the management of instruments which are heat sensitive, and when time pressures influence the process chosen:

- Formaldehyde—a carcinogenic solution which should only be used in controlled situations, such as the sealed environment of low temperature steam and formaldehyde sterilization units.
- Glutaraldehyde or buffered peracetic acid—stringent health and safety measures must be in place for the use of this acidic solution; protocols must be strictly adhered to. This is generally the agent of choice when time influences the process.

Hydrogen peroxide plasma sterilization

This system reduces or eliminates the use of the liquid disinfectants. It can be used to track equipment and is suitable for both metallic and nonmetallic instruments. This system also reduces the risk of spillage and the dangers associated with inhalation from liquid disinfectants.

4   CREUTZFELDT-JAKOB DISEASE

This topic must be addressed in relation to instrumentation and the procedures to be adopted within the OR if patients are confirmed as having Creutzfeldt-Jakob disease (CJD) or suspected in any way.

First recognized in 1921, CJD is one of several transmissible spongiform encephalopathies which affect both animals and humans [6].

CJD may present in three ways:

- Sporadic—this form is not yet fully understood, but several theories suggest that this will be proved to be environmental in origin.
- Genetic—this stems from an inherited defect or mutation of the gene which encodes for normal prion protein, possibly triggered around 50–60 years of age.
- Acquired—this is triggered by contamination with an infected agent or abnormal prion disease. One route is via contaminated instruments [7].

When surgery is necessary, it is important to ascertain which tissues will be operated on.

Tissue can be divided into three risk categories:

- High—this includes the brain, spinal cord and posterior eye.
- Medium—including the anterior eye and olfactory epithelium, and also lymphoid tissue.
- Low—all remaining body tissues.

It is very important for the ORP involved with spine surgery to have an insight into the subject of CJD. This will enable the team to assess the risk and apply the appropriate precautions in line with departmental policy.

Dyke [6] sets out points to run alongside strict universal precautions. These are:

- Only use single-use spinal and epidural sets.
- Use single-use instruments whenever possible.
- Never attempt to reuse single-use equipment.
- Set tracking systems for instruments if they are not currently in place.
- Mandatory tracking systems for endoscopes.
- Avoid using power tools (prevent error of reuse).
- Follow protocols.
- Have a one-way flow of instruments.
- Known or suspected cases should be done at the end of the list.
- Have a minimal number of staff in the OR.

4.1   PREPARATION, QUARANTINE, AND DISPOSAL OF INSTRUMENTS

Single-use instruments should be used wherever available and practicable, without compromising the surgical outcome of the patient. However, this may be difficult due to the limited amount and range of instruments available, particularly with regard to power tools and attachments.

If the patient is considered to be in the high or medium risk category all instruments and equipment used must be disposed of by incineration. If the patient is classed as low risk the instruments can be recycled according to individual units' best practice guidelines.

Impervious plastic containers with tight fitting lids for disposal of instrumentation must be available at the end of any procedure. Containers should be clearly labeled with details of the contents, date, OR, and contact number. If instruments are to be quarantined until the risk status has been clarified, then the instruments should be retained as above where the equipment is stored and again clearly marked. Most importantly, the room or storage area must be kept locked at all times, eliminating the risk of reuse.

---

5 BIBLIOGRAPHY

1. **Clarke P, Jones J** (1998) *Brigden's Operating Department Practice.* Edingburgh: Churchill Livingston.
2. **Line S** (2003) Decontamination and control of infection in theatre. *Br J Perioper Nurs;* 13(2):70–75.
3. **McGeough M** (2001) Sterilisation and traceability of surgical instruments. *Br J Perioper Nurs;* 11(10):434.
4. **Miller J** (2002) Instrument reprocessing in theatres. *Br J Perioper Nurs;* 12(1):34–38.
5. **Hewitson P** (2000) Decontamination and the law. A better understanding. *Br J Perioper Nurs;* 10(8):405–411.
6. **Dyke M** (2001) Creutzfeldt-Jakob disease. The story so far. *Br J Perioper Nurs;* 11(2):64–68.
7. **McNeil B** (2004) Management of a CJD case. Part 1. Preoperative organization of the case. *Br J Perioper Nurs;* 14(4):164–170.

3.6   SURGICAL APPROACHES TO THE SPINE

1   ANTERIOR APPROACH TO THE CERVICAL SPINE

The cervical spine can be approached in many different ways. Common approaches utilized are:

- transoral,
- submandibular,
- anterolateral,
- lateral, or
- anteromedial.

The most common approach to the subaxial cervical spine (C3–7) is via the anteromedial approach. This is utilized to address fractures, tumors, degenerative stenosis, disc herniations, and infections.

The anteromedial approach starts with a transverse skin incision from the midline extending laterally. A vertical incision may be used for exposure of multiple levels. The right- or left-sided approach depends on the surgeon's preference. Some surgeons prefer the left-sided approach because the location of

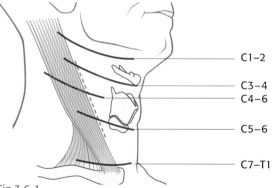

Fig 3.6-1
The approximate skin incision for specific spinal levels usually corresponds with palpable subcutaneous structures. C1–2 lies under the angle of the jaw, C3–4 a centimeter above the thyroid cartilage in the region of the hyoid bone, C4–5 at the level of the thyroid cartilage, C5–6 at the cricoid cartilage, and C7–T1 in the supraclavicular area.

the recurrent laryngeal nerve is more predictable in the tracheoesophageal groove.

The level of incision is based on surface anatomy that corresponds to the intended spinal level (**Fig 3.6-1**).

After the skin incision, the subcutaneous tissue is undermined with scissors to allow mobilization of the skin. Superficial retractors are placed. The platysma muscle is incised in line with the skin incision. Deep to the platysma, the external and anterior jugular veins may need to be ligated.

The key landmark to this approach is the sternocleidomastoid (SCM) muscle (**Fig 3.6-2**).

The medial border of the SCM is dissected free with scissors, peanut, or finger. Blunt dissection, medial to the SCM and lateral to the strap muscles, goes directly towards the spine. Angled retractors may be used to aid visualization. The middle cervical fascia is incised just medial to the carotid sheath (**Fig 3.6-3**).

Blunt dissection extends the interval superiorly and inferiorly. This opens up access to the spine.

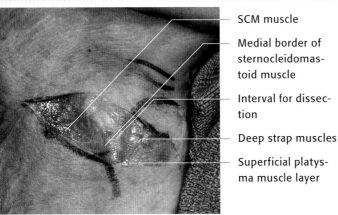

- SCM muscle
- Medial border of sternocleidomastoid muscle
- Interval for dissection
- Deep strap muscles
- Superficial platysma muscle layer

Fig 3.6-2
The interval for dissection is medial to the SCM muscle and lateral to the strap muscles.

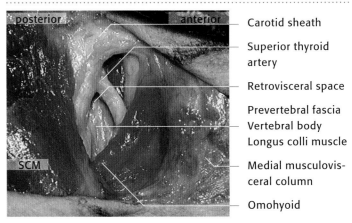

posterior   anterior
- Carotid sheath
- Superior thyroid artery
- Retrovisceral space
- Prevertebral fascia
- Vertebral body
- Longus colli muscle
- Medial musculovisceral column
- Omohyoid

SCM

Fig 3.6-3
The interval for dissection continues medial to the carotid sheath and lateral to the trachea and esophagus, down to the prevertebral fascia and spine.

2   ANTERIOR APPROACH TO THE THORACIC SPINE

A deep retractor, such as a Cloward, is used to retract the SCM and carotid sheath laterally and the strap muscles, trachea, and esophagus medially. The longus colli muscle is incised in the midline and elevated laterally with electrocautery, peanut, or elevator. The Cloward retractor can be inserted deep to the elevated longus colli muscle (**Fig 3.6-4**).

A marker needle is inserted in the disc and a lateral x-ray is taken to ensure the appropriate level. At this time, the definitive surgery is performed.

The thoracic spine is approached anteriorly by removing a rib. Surgeon preference determines which rib is removed. The rib corresponding to the caudal vertebral body is often used to approach a disc space. For example, the 9th rib attaches at the T8–9 disc space. A left-sided approach is preferable because the aorta is easier to mobilize than the inferior vena cava. This places the patient in the right lateral decubitus position.

The skin incision is made along the course of the rib to be removed (**Fig 3.6-5**).

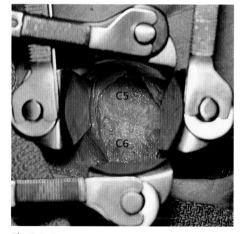

Fig 3.6-4
Insertion of the Cloward retractor allows visualization and access to the vertebral bodies and discs.

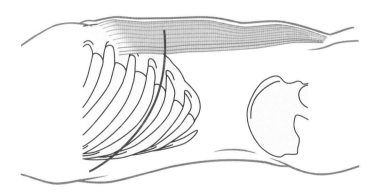

Fig 3.6-5
The skin incision made from the lateral border of the paraspinous musculature to the sternocostal junction over the rib to be removed.

Posteriorly, the incision begins lateral to the paraspinous muscles and continues anteriorly to the costochondral junction. Once the subcutaneous tissues are divided, superficial retractors are positioned. Using electrocautery, the muscle layers of the thorax are divided down to the rib. The periosteum is incised with electrocautery and elevated off the bone with a Cobb or curved-tip periosteal elevator. The periosteum is circumferentially stripped off the bone with a Doyen or Cobb elevator (**Fig 3.6-6**).

The rib is cut at the costochondral junction, lifted with a Kocher, elevated and cut posteriorly between the costotransverse joint and angle of the rib. Any sharp edges of the rib stump are smoothed with a rasp or rongeur and bone wax is applied.

The rib bed is incised with forceps and scissors (**Fig 3.6-7**).

The undersurface of the rib bed and parietal pleura is cleared free of any pleural adhesions. The lung is protected by the surgeon's hand or sponge stick while the incision in the rib bed and pleura is extended with semi-closed scissors. The Fenochetti rib retractor is placed with a wet sponge on either side. A lung retractor may also be used.

The view of the spine at this point is obscured by the parietal pleura as it covers the soft-tissue structures over the spinal column (**Fig 3.6-8**).

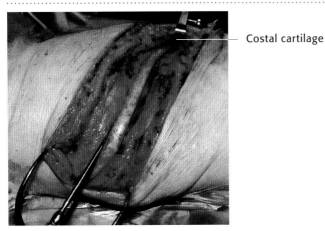

Costal cartilage

Fig 3.6-6
The periosteum is circumferentially stripped off the rib with a Doyen or Cobb elevator.

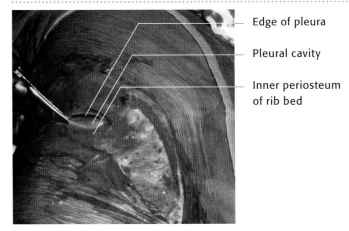

Edge of pleura

Pleural cavity

Inner periosteum of rib bed

Fig 3.6-7
The rib bed is incised with forceps and scissors exposing the pleural cavity.

An incision in the pleura directly over a disc space is made with forceps and scissors. The discs are identified as the "hills" and the vertebral bodies are the "valleys".

The underlying vessels and soft tissues are dissected free from the pleura with a peanut as the pleural incision is extended cephalad and caudad. Segmental vessels lying in the valley of the vertebral bodies (**Fig 3.6-9**) are dissected free with a right-angle clamp and either ligated with 2–0 suture or cauterized. Elevation of the pleura off the anterior aspect of the spinal column is performed with peanuts, Cobb elevators, and/or swabs.

At this point, exposure of the spinal column is complete and the procedure of choice is performed. The rib head may be removed in order to gain access to the posterior disc and spinal canal.

Closure begins with permanent braided suture for the parietal pleura covering the spine. A chest tube is inserted. The rib approximator closes the thoracotomy site. The rib bed and overlying muscle layers are closed with suture. The subcutaneous tissue and skin are closed as the surgeon desires.

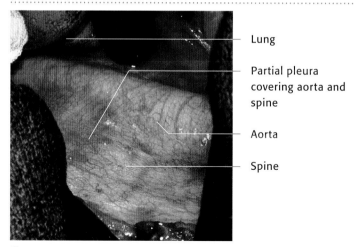

Lung

Partial pleura covering aorta and spine

Aorta

Spine

Fig 3.6-8
The parietal pleura covers the aorta and spine.

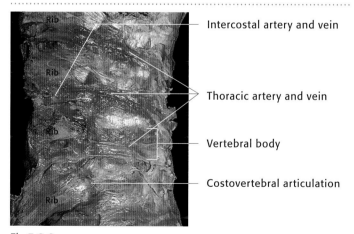

Intercostal artery and vein

Thoracic artery and vein

Vertebral body

Costovertebral articulation

Fig 3.6-9
The intercostal vessels lie in the middle of the vertebral body and continue along the inferior aspect of the rib.

3   ANTERIOR APPROACH TO THE THORACOLUMBAR SPINE

The anterior thoracolumbar approach is most commonly used for either an anterior release and fusion or instrumentation and correction for thoracolumbar scoliosis. The patient is positioned in the lateral decubitus with the convex side of the curve facing up. The surgeon chooses which rib to resect to gain access. Resection of the ninth rib provides exposure from T11–12 and distal, therefore, will be described in this chapter.

The skin is incised directly over the ninth rib. Posteriorly, the incision starts lateral to the paraspinous muscles, it continues anteriorly to the costochondral junction where it curves distally along the lateral border of the rectus sheath (**Fig 3.6-10**). Once the subcutaneous tissues are divided, superficial retractors are placed. The muscle layers of the thorax are divided with electrocautery down to the rib. The periosteum over the ninth rib is incised with electrocautery and elevated off the bone with a Cobb elevator or curved-tip periosteal elevator. The periosteum is circumferentially stripped off the bone with a Doyen or Cobb elevator. The rib is cut at the costochondral junction, lifted with a Kocher, and cut posteriorly between the costotransverse joint and angle of the rib. Any sharp edges of the rib stump are smoothed with a rasp or rongeur and bone wax is applied.

The rib bed is incised with forceps and scissors. The undersurface of the rib bed and parietal pleura is cleared free of any pleural adhesions. The lung is protected by the surgeon's hand

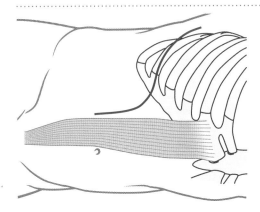

Fig 3.6-10
The incision starts lateral to the paraspinous muscles, it continues anteriorly over the rib to be removed to the costochondral junction where it curves distally along the lateral border of the rectus sheath.

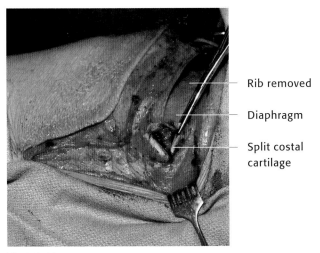

Rib removed

Diaphragm

Split costal cartilage

Fig 3.6-11
After incising the rib bed, the costal cartilage is split in half.

or sponge stick while the incision in the rib bed and pleura is extended with semi-closed scissors.

Anteriorly, the costal cartilage is split in half and tagged with suture (**Fig 3.6-11**).

The retroperitoneal fat is identified deep to the cartilage (**Fig 3.6-12**).

After the undersurface of the costal cartilage is bluntly dissected free of any peritoneal attachments, the incision is continued through the cartilage caudally just lateral to the rectus sheath.

The surgeon follows the retroperitoneal fat laterally, bluntly dissecting the peritoneum off the inferior surface of the diaphragm. Peanuts, sponge stick, or finger dissection may be used for this maneuver. The peritoneum is also dissected off the transversalis fascia and abdominal wall caudally. With the peritoneum retracted, the abdominal musculature (external oblique, internal oblique, and transversus abdominis) is incised just lateral to the rectus sheath.

A Fenochetti rib retractor is placed in the defect of the thorax with a wet sponge on either side. A lung retractor may also be used. The diaphragm is incised 2 cm from its lateral edge, starting anteriorly and curving posteriorly (**Fig 3.6-13**). 2–0 tag sutures are used for later reapproximation.

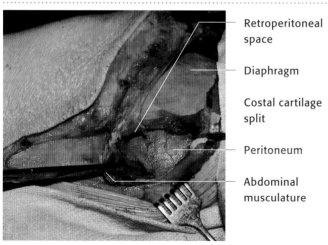

Retroperitoneal space

Diaphragm

Costal cartilage split

Peritoneum

Abdominal musculature

Fig 3.6-12
The retroperitoneal space is located deep to the split costal cartilage.

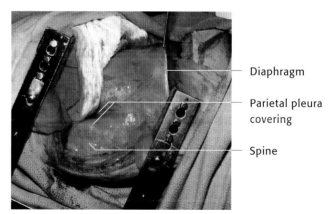

Diaphragm

Parietal pleura covering

Spine

Fig 3.6-13
The diaphragm is incised 2 cm from its lateral attachment.

An incision in the pleura is made with forceps and scissors. The underlying vessels and soft tissues are dissected free from the pleura with a peanut as the pleural incision is extended cephalad and caudad. Segmental vessels lying in the valley of the vertebral bodies are dissected free with a right-angle clamp and either ligated with 2–0 suture or cauterized. Elevation of the pleura off the anterior aspect of the spinal column is performed with peanuts, Cobb elevators, and/or swabs (**Fig 3.6-14**).

The crus of the diaphragm is identified by the transverse muscle fibers attaching to the spine at L1, L2, and L3. The crus is dissected off the spine with electrocautery as the peritoneum is retracted anteriorly with a Deavor retractor. The psoas muscle is also dissected off the lumbar spine to provide visualization.

The thoracolumbar spine is now exposed, allowing the appropriate procedure to be performed.

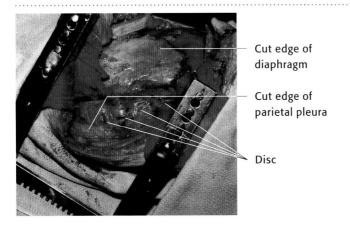

Cut edge of diaphragm

Cut edge of parietal pleura

Disc

Fig 3.6-14
Elevation of the pleura off the spine exposes the vertebral bodies (valleys) and discs (hills). The intercostal vessels lie on the vertebral bodies.

4   ANTERIOR APPROACH TO THE LUMBAR SPINE

The skin incision is made 1 cm left of the midline. To approach L4–5, the incision starts just distal to the umbilicus and descends 6 cm caudally. To approach L5–S1, the incision is the middle third of the distance between the umbilicus and pubis.

Alternatively, the skin incision may be made transversely or obliquely (**Fig 3.6-15**).

The dissection proceeds through the subcutaneous tissue to the anterior rectus sheath. Superficial retractors are placed in the wound. Bleeding vessels are picked up with forceps and coagulated with electrocautery.

The anterior rectus sheath is incised with a scalpel 1 cm lateral to its medial border. The incision is extended cephalad and caudad with scissors. Two Langenbeck retractors are placed deep to the rectus muscle for the assistant to retract laterally. Vessels are electrocauterized.

The surgeon identifies the arcuate line, which is the inferior margin of the posterior rectus sheath. Distal to the arcuate line, the surgeon picks up the transversalis fascia with forceps. The assistant picks up the transversalis fascia near the surgeon's hold to allow the surgeon to incise a small hole in the fascia. A peanut dissects off the underlying peritoneum from the fascia. Soft-tissue holders are used to pick up more and

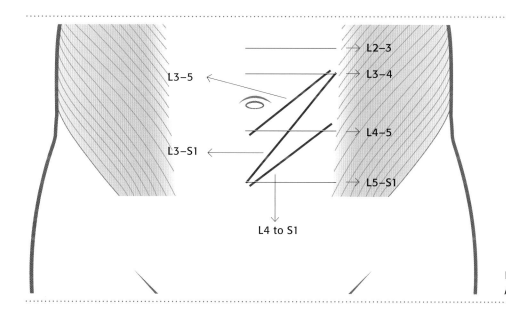

Fig 3.6-15
Area for skin incisions.

more of the fascia as peritoneum is dissected free. The fascia is incised proximally to the arcuate line. Once peritoneum is dissected free from the undersurface of the posterior rectus sheath, the arcuate line is incised proximally.

The direction of the dissection changes towards inferior and lateral. Peritoneum is peeled off the transversalis fascia working towards the fat in the inferior and lateral corner (**Fig 3.6-16**). When around the lateral aspect of peritoneum, the peritoneum and abdominal contents are swept medially (**Fig 3.6-17**).

Adhesions may need to be released proximally to allow completion of this maneuver. The psoas muscle is located deep to the peritoneum, positioned just lateral to the spine. Identification of the iliac vessels anterior to the spine is essential. Peritoneum is mobilized over the psoas muscle and iliac vessels to the contralateral side of the spine. The retractor blades are inserted at this point.

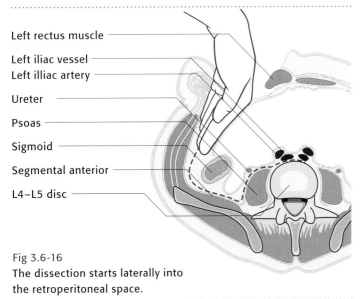

Left rectus muscle

Left iliac vessel

Left illiac artery

Ureter

Psoas

Sigmoid

Segmental anterior

L4–L5 disc

Fig 3.6-16
The dissection starts laterally into the retroperitoneal space.

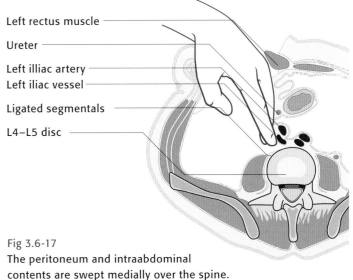

Left rectus muscle

Ureter

Left illiac artery

Left iliac vessel

Ligated segmentals

L4–L5 disc

Fig 3.6-17
The peritoneum and intraabdominal contents are swept medially over the spine.

The appropriate disc level is visualized by clearing off soft tissue with peanuts. The assistant picks up bleeding vessels with forceps and electrocautery. Care must be taken not to damage the superior hypogastric plexus of sympathetic nerves located just distal to the aortic bifurcation and anterior to the L5 vertebral body. Some surgeons prefer bipolar cautery in this area, however, as little cautery as possible is essential to preserve the sympathetic nerves.

For exposure of the L5–S1 disc, the median sacral vessels are usually electrocauterized (**Fig 3.6-18**).

For exposure of the L4–L5 disc, the iliolumbar vein located inferior and to the left of the left iliac vein may have to be ligated (**Fig 3.6-19**).

The indicated procedure is performed at this point.

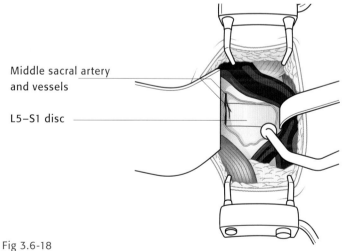

Middle sacral artery and vessels

L5–S1 disc

Fig 3.6-18
Sacrificing the median sacral vessels and mobilizing the left iliac vein and artery laterally exposes the L5–S1 disc space.

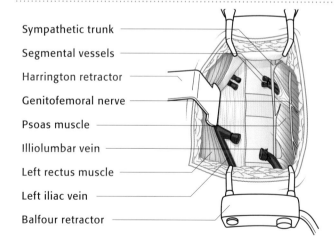

Sympathetic trunk

Segmental vessels

Harrington retractor

Genitofemoral nerve

Psoas muscle

Illiolumbar vein

Left rectus muscle

Left iliac vein

Balfour retractor

Fig 3.6-19
The iliolumbar vein may need to be ligated in order to mobilize the iliac vessels to the right side of the spine for exposure of the L4–5 disc.

5   POSTERIOR APPROACH TO THE CERVICAL SPINE

A midline incision is made through the skin. Superficial retractors are placed in the wound. Tension on the wound edges allows the surgeon to cut down along the white median raphe with either a scalpel or electrocautery. The raphe takes a circuitous route, rarely a straight line. Cutting along the avascular raphe avoids the paraspinous muscle, thereby, decreasing blood loss.

Dissection is carried down to the spinous processes. The spinous processes of C2 to C6 are identified by their bifid shape. Subperiosteal dissection down the spinous process, along the lamina, and out to the lateral edge of the lateral mass is performed with a Cobb elevator and electrocautery. Deep retractors are placed.

The posterior arch of C1 will be deep compared to the spinous process of C2. Subperiosteal dissection of the posterior arch of C1 is carried out with a Cobb elevator and electrocautery. The surgeon should limit exposure to 1.5 cm lateral to the midline to avoid the vertebral artery (**Fig 3.6-20**).

The second cervical ganglion is a useful landmark as it lies in the groove for the vertebral artery.

To enter the spinal canal, a Zielke rongeur removes the midline interspinous ligament. Dissection is carried down to the yellow ligamentum flavum, which can also be removed with a Zielke rongeur. Once the superficial midline structures are sufficiently removed, epidural fat will become visible. At this point, a Kerrison rongeur removes the ligamentum flavum from medial to lateral. Immediately deep to the ligamentum flavum and epidural fat is the dura surrounding the spinal cord.

At this point, the surgeon will finish the procedure of choice.

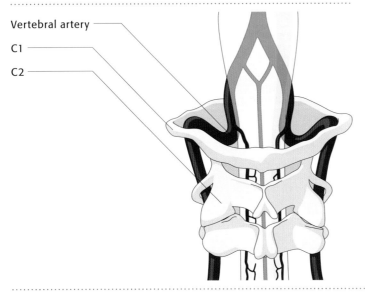

Vertebral artery

C1

C2

Fig 3.6-20
In the subaxial cervical spine, the vertebral artery runs anterior to the facet joints. More cephalad, the vertebral artery sits in a relatively exposed position just lateral to the C1–2 articulation.

6   POSTERIOR APPROACH TO THE THORACIC SPINE

A straight midline incision is made through the skin. Dissection with scalpel or electrocautery is performed through the subcutaneous tissue down to the posterior thoracic fascia. Superficial retractors are placed in the wound. Subcutaneous fat may be stripped off the fascia with a Cobb elevator to facilitate closure. Bleeding vessels are electrocauterized.

The posterior thoracic fascia is incised in the midline. Subperiosteal dissection with a Cobb elevator and electrocautery is performed down the spinous process and out laterally along the lamina and facet joint. A swab is placed in the dissected cavity. The surgeon repeats the step at the next level until all the indicated levels are dissected. A deep retractor is placed to retract the paraspinous muscle. Subperiosteal dissection is continued over the transverse process at each level.

At this point, the surgeon may proceed with a decompression procedure. A Zielke rongeur removes the midline interspinous ligament. Dissection is carried down to the yellow ligamentum flavum, which can also be removed with a Zielke rongeur. Once the superficial midline structures are sufficiently removed, epidural fat will become visible. A Kerrison rongeur removes the ligamentum flavum from medial to lateral. Immediately deep to the ligamentum flavum and epidural fat is the dura surrounding the spinal cord.

Alternatively, a costotransversectomy may be performed. In this situation, the surgeon removes the rib head and transverse process in order to gain access to the lateral and anterior aspect of the vertebral body. Subperiosteal dissection is performed along the transverse process, rib head, and medial 3 cm of rib. The periosteum is stripped circumferentially off the medial 4 cm of rib with a small Cobb elevator. A swab is used to protect the pleura. The rib is cut 3 cm lateral to the rib head. The rib head is removed with a rat-tooth rongeur (**Fig 3.6-21**).

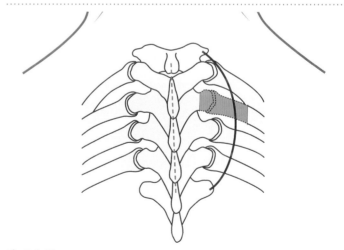

Fig 3.6-21
The transverse process, rib head, and medial 3 cm of rib are removed for lateral access to the spine.

The intercostals vessels located inferior to the rib are ligated or cauterized. The pleura is bluntly dissected off the rib head and vertebral body with a peanut. This allows access to the lateral and anterior spine.

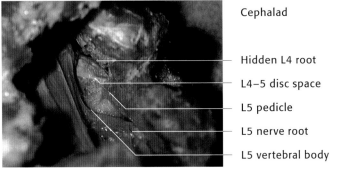

Fig 3.6-22
Preservation of the pars interarticularis and the facet joint lateral to the medial wall of the pedicle is essential to preserve stability.

Cephalad

Hidden L4 root

L4–5 disc space

L5 pedicle

L5 nerve root

L5 vertebral body

7   POSTERIOR APPROACH TO THE LUMBAR SPINE

A midline incision is made in the skin. Dissection through the subcutaneous tissue with scalpel or electrocautery is performed down to the posterior lumbar fascia. Superficial retractors are placed in the wound. Subcutaneous fat may be stripped off the fascia with a Cobb elevator to facilitate closure. Bleeding vessels are electrocauterized.

The fascia is incised with electrocautery. Subperiosteal dissection with a Cobb elevator is carried down the spinous process, out the lamina to the facet joints. Deep retractors are placed. A Cobb elevator peels tissue and muscle attachments off the facet joint capsules, preserving the joints if needed. A rat-tooth rongeur removes tissue from the interlaminar area and pars interarticularis. The assistant can be very helpful by anticipating bleeding vessels at the pars interarticularis at this point. The vessels are electrocauterized with forceps. The dissection may be extended laterally around the facet joints and down to the transverse processes if a fusion is planned.

There are a variety of techniques to decompress the lumbar spine. Commonly, a rat-tooth rongeur removes superficial soft tissue and potentially bone from the spinous process and lamina. A curette may be utilized to locate the cephalad edge of the caudal lamina and to detach the ligamentum flavum. A Kerrison rongeur is used to remove the ligamentum flavum and to perform a laminotomy. A laminotomy is the removal of bone from the cephalad or caudal lamina in order to enlarge the exposure of neural elements. A laminectomy entails removal of the entire lamina. The surgeon removes the necessary amount of bone and soft tissue in order to visualize and decompress the neural tissue. Preservation of the pars interarticularis and the facet joint lateral to the medial wall of the pedicle is essential to preserve stability (**Fig 3.6-22**).

8   SUGGESTIONS FOR FURTHER READING

Bohlman HH, Eismont FJ (1981) Surgical techniques of anterior decompression and fusion for spinal cord injuries. *Clin Orthop;* 154:57–67.

Bridwell KH, DeWald RL, Hammerberg KW, et al (1997) *The Textbook of Spinal Surgery.* 2nd ed. Philadelphia: JB Lippincott Company.

Herkowitz HN, Rothman RH, Simeone FA (1999) *Rothman-Simeone: the Spine.* 4th ed. Philadelphia: W.B. Saunders Company.

Hodgson AR, Yau ACMC (1964) *Anterior surgical approaches to the spinal column.* Apley AG (ed): Recent Advances in Orthopaedics. Baltimore: Williams & Wilkins, 289–323.

Robinson RA, Southwick WO (1960) *Surgical approaches to the cervical spine.* American Academy of Orthopaedic Surgery: Instructional Course Lectures, Vol XVII. St. Louis: Mosby, 229–330.

Watkins RG (2003) *Surgical Approaches to the Spine.* 2nd ed. New York: Springer-Verlag.

Sue Corbett, Michele Goodwin, Angela Hallworth, Hayley Johnson, Ruth Knight, Helen Nelson, Carmel Nosworthy, Janine Roulston, Toni Swaby, Sue Ward, Christina Zarifova

3 OPERATIVE KNOWLEDGE FOR SPINE SURGERY

3.7 IMMEDIATE POSTOPERATIVE CARE

1 INTRODUCTION

This chapter addresses immediate postoperative care for the spinal patient in relation to operating room (OR) recovery. It is useful to consider both the medical and holistic care the patient will receive postoperatively before returning to the ward.

We can look at this care in terms of seven primary areas of management:

- airway management,
- acute pain management,
- nausea and vomiting,
- neurological assessments,
- peripheral drainage care,
- skin and pressure area care,
- emotional and psychological support.

2 AIRWAY MANAGEMENT

On arrival in the OR recovery the patient will still be under the influence of anesthesia, and therefore the immediate focus is to maintain the patient's airway. The prescribed amount of oxygen will be delivered via a face mask.

Airway management is the most important role of the recovery nurse, as respiratory problems, including hypoxia, are the commonest form of postoperative death and injury. Postoperative hypoxia increases the rate of cell damage to the relevant organs. The signs include:

- confusion,
- restlessness,
- aggression,
- agitation,
- deterioration–mental state,
- level of consciousness [1].

Following spine surgery it may be necessary for the patient to be kept supine and to some degree immobile. The administration of oxygen is important to prevent hypoxia, recognizable by the above signs. If the patient experiences symptoms of hypoxia, extra care must be taken to prevent dislodgement of any surgical drains, as this may lead to unnecessary postoperative complications, which may involve a return to the OR for further wound exploration.

Continuous monitoring of the pulse and blood pressure to assess cardiovascular stability and adequate oxygenation is of high importance. Careful observation of the lips and fingernails must also be made, to detect any symptoms of cyanosis.

Postoperative airway complications are common to some degree, and the two main causes are:

- Airway obstruction—caused by the tongue, resulting from the contraction of the pharyngeal muscles, swelling, or blood/secretions collecting in the pharynx [2]. Airway problems are detected by continuous assessment of the rate, depth, and rhythm of breathing and the detection of air moving in and out of the mouth.
- Laryngeal spasm—may be partial or complete, caused by stimulation of the cords by blood/secretions, or the type of airway used. It is characterized by noisy breathing.

Airway obstruction can be corrected simply by patient stimulation. Basic airway management skills can be utilized in the form of head tilt or chin lift. This raises the tongue from the pharynx, which alleviates the obstruction. Applying these techniques when the patient has undergone cervical surgery, however, must be undertaken with care.

3   ACUTE PAIN MANAGEMENT

The type of pain experienced by the spinal patient is acute pain. It is short in duration, and linked to the time of healing. The International Association for the Study of Pain (IASP) identified pain as an unpleasant sensory and emotional experience associated with actual or potential tissue damage [3].

3.1   NATURE OF PAIN

The perception of pain is a function of the sensory nervous system. Pain is sensed by nociceptors, which exist throughout almost all body tissue, especially the skin. The nociceptors may be stimulated by mechanical, thermal, or chemical changes. If the stimulus is of sufficient magnitude, an electrical impulse will be generated and transmitted along the sensory nerve fiber to the posterior horn of the spinal cord. There, the primary afferent neurone synapses with the secondary neurone and the message travels towards the brain via the spinothalamic tract [4].

3.2   EFFECTS OF SURGERY

A surgical procedure presents an enormous insult to nociceptive pathways. High levels of stimulation can cause changes that result in hypersensitivity, which means normally nonnoxious stimuli (such as touch) can produce pain, a phenomenon known as allodynia. In addition, the amplitude and duration of painful stimulus increases a phenomenon known as hyperalgesia. The full affect is known as central sensitization. These effects mean any painful stimulus has a greater chance of being transmitted to the brain and recognized as pain. Small doses of opioid administered before the stimulus occurs can suppress hyperalgesia, whereas much larger doses of opioid are required to achieve the same response once hyperalgesia has been established by the surgical procedure [5]. An understanding of these factors provides a rationale for early and aggressive pain management.

Acute pain activates the sympathetic nervous system, causing a number of physiological stress responses to promote healing, fight infection, prevent further damage and minimize blood loss.

In unrelieved acute pain, a variety of harmful effects may occur:

- Cardiovascular system—tachycardia, increased cardiac output, hypertension, myocardial ischemia, myocardial infarction, hypercoagulation, deep vein thrombosis, and increased peripheral vascular resistance.
- Respiratory system—increased respiratory rate, reduced ability to breathe deeply, atelectasis, shunting, and sputum retention.
- Depression of the immune system—increased metabolism, glucose intolerance, and hyperglycemia.
- Gastrointestinal system—ileus and decreased gastric emptying.
- Endocrine system—increased adrenocorticotrophic hormone, angiotensin II, antidiuretic hormone, aldosterone, catecholamines, cortisol, and epinephrine.
- Genitourinary system—decreased urinary output, urinary retention, fluid overload, and hypokalemia.
- Musculoskeletal system—muscle spasm, impaired muscle function, fatigue, and skeletal muscle breakdown.
- Sympathetic nervous system—increased adrenaline, and noradrenaline.
- Psychological and cognitive effects—sleeplessness anxiety, fear, disorientation, reduction in cognitive function, and mental confusion [6].

3.3   PAIN ASSESSMENT

The working party of the commission on the provision of surgical services concluded in 1990 that pain cannot be treated if it is not assessed on a regular basis, thus pain assessment is vital upon admission and throughout the patient's stay in hospital.

Patient characteristics that impact on pain control:

- Premorbid pain status—opioid exposure, concomitant therapy.
- Degree of pain—mild, moderate, severe.
- Comorbidities-metabolic, cardiovascular, GI, kidney/liver, CNS.
- Expectations of pain and pain control.
- Age, gender, ethnicity, mental status, addictive behavior.
- Degree of invasiveness or tissue damage—mild, moderate.
- Physiological source of pain—somatic, visceral, neuropathic.
- Expected length of stay in hospital—outpatient, inpatient.

Misconceptions about pain and realistic expectations in relation to pain relief should be discussed.

Pain measurement

Preoperative education for the patient about the pain measurement tool, the goals of pain assessment, and the patient's role in the assessment process is necessary. If pain is to be managed effectively it is vital to use a pain assessment tool; this provides documented evidence of the efficacy or failure of any of the drugs, reduces the chances of bias and error, and helps communication with other professionals. Therefore, it is necessary to identify a simple pain tool to measure pain intensity, such as verbal descriptors (eg, none, mild, moderate, and severe) on the numerical scale (0–10), 0 = no pain, 10 = severe pain. This tool is quickly and easily understood.

Important considerations are:

- Frequency of pain measurement—this should be done frequently and should take into account operation type, pain severity, analgesic regimen and any change in the analgesic regimen.
- Pain measurements should be in the patient's own words where at all possible. "Pain is whatever the person experiencing it says it is, and it occurs whenever the person experiencing it says it does" [6].
- Pain measurement should assess the effect of pain treatments when at rest, during deep breathing, coughing, and other activities.
- Pain measurement should always be documented alongside the intervention undertaken.
- Uncontrolled or unexpected pain should indicate further clinical examination.

3.4   PHARMACOLOGICAL INTERVENTIONS IN ACUTE SPINAL PAIN MANAGEMENT

Acute pain is characterized by signs of hyperactivity in the autonomic nervous system, such as sweating and vasoconstriction. It responds well to analgesic therapy and treatment of the underlying cause of pain [5]. Evidence suggests that patients benefit from the use of multimodal analgesia, eg, opioids, nonsteroidal anti-inflammatory drugs (NSAID), paracetamol, and local anesthetics.

Preemptive analgesia to prevent changes in the spinal cord that occur with repetitive input of painful stimuli from the site of injury, which may lead to an exaggerated response to pain is still inconsistent [7], but further research is required.

The analgesic ladder may be used in reverse to guide analgesic strengths in acute spinal pain:

1. Pain + nonopioid ± adjuvant.
2. Pain persisting or increasing. Opioid for mild to moderate pain + nonopioid + adjuvant.
3. Pain persisting or increasing. Opioid for moderate to severe pain ± nonopioid + adjuvant. Freedom from pain [8].

Morphine

Morphine is the most powerful analgesic available and is viewed as the gold standard of pain relief. It produces analgesia by binding to opioid receptors which are found in the brain and spinal cord. There are three different types of opioid receptors: mu, kappa, and delta receptors. Morphine acts on the mu receptors which can result in the side effects such as respiratory depression, nausea, and a decrease in conscious level [9]. Many nurses believe that the administration of opioids postoperatively compromises a patient's respiratory function, however, under medication with opioids will result in increased pain and is more likely to cause respiratory difficulties. Side effects are reversible, eg, use of the antagonist naloxone [5].

Patient-controlled analgesia

Generally, patient-controlled analgesia has been associated with better pain relief and greater patient satisfaction compared to intermittent opioid injections. Peaks and troughs associated with the larger doses given by intramuscular administration are thus avoided, helping to prevent side effects. Patient-controlled analgesia was very good in clinical trials, indicating that when good advice and education is given to the patient, improved pain management is achieved.

Nonsteroidal anti-inflammatory drugs (NSAID)

NSAID work by inhibiting an enzyme called cyclooxygenase, which is responsible for the production of prostaglandin. By inhibiting prostaglandin production, pain intensity is decreased. Unfortunately, one of the downsides of these drugs is their ability to block all cyclooxygenase enzymes. These include those enzymes needed for the production of the mucosa that protects the stomach and small intestine, as well as the chemicals that maintain renal function and platelet adhesion. NSAID are effective in the management of acute postoperative spinal pain, especially in combination with opioids. They may also lead to a 20–40% reduction in opioid requirement [7]. Adverse events include increased coagulation time, and renal failure, which can be precipitated in patients with preexisting heart or kidney disease.

Paracetamol

Paracetamol increases the effectiveness of other analgesics and can be given as an adjunct to an opioid for more severe pain.

Regional neural blockade

The use of local anesthesia given in a single dose is common practice. It provides pain relief postoperatively in the first few hours, thus making further pain relief unnecessary [7]. It may be used when an epidural is contraindicated, eg, at risk of spinal hematomas.

Nurses, surgeons, anesthetists, and the patients themselves share the responsibility for achieving optimal pain relief postoperatively.

4   NAUSEA AND VOMITING

It is suggested that the incidence of postoperative nausea and vomiting is as high as 56–92% [10], which indicates that this is still a significant postoperative complication.

The most significant risk to the patient undergoing any type of surgery continues to be that of vomiting under anesthesia, leading to aspiration pneumonitis, esophageal rupture, and alveolar rupture, leading to airway compromise. Other complications include obstruction, anoxia, and potential brain damage. This has led to a traditional six-hour preoperative fasting protocol (food and fluids) for all patients undergoing anesthesia or sedation. This has recently been reviewed in the case of shorter surgical procedures, based on research by Brady et al [11], which concluded that it was sufficient to withhold food, but allow fluids up to a few hours preoperatively, because this did not adversely influence postoperative nausea and vomiting.

The nausea and vomiting process is multifactorial, based on complex physiology, and as such, a holistic structured approach to treatment is advantageous in improving outcomes.

The body has an excellent distribution of both mechanoreceptors and baroreceptors which respond to minute pressure and chemical changes in the body which are an inevitable part of the anesthetic and surgical process. Various nerve pathways link up with these receptor sites, and the information is transmitted by neurotransmitters such as acetylcholine, dopamine, histamine, and 5-hydroxytryptamine.

There are many factors which precipitate vomiting:

- anxiety,
- gender—females are more susceptible,
- history of previous sickness,
- length of surgery,
- choice of drugs,
- oxygenation and hydration,
- pain,
- medical or surgical history of obstruction or laparoscopic procedures,
- unanticipated cardiac events,
- use of opioids.

Regardless of history or gender, the patient undergoing major spine surgery will almost certainly be susceptible to postoperative nausea and vomiting, because of the lengthy procedures involved requiring large amounts of drugs, including a considerable amount of opiates both intraoperatively and postoperatively.

The choice of drugs given in anesthesia affects outcome considerably. Hydration is a factor, but it is not always possible to control this perfectly in spine surgery where there is potential for bleeding.

Vomiting can also cause bleeding or disruption of the surgery, so for this reason should be avoided if at all possible. Although anti-inflammatory steroidal drugs are less emetic, they are not suitable for spine surgery because of their tendency to increase bleeding. For this reason, the use of opiates is often impossible to avoid, even though they may contribute to vomiting.

The effective management of this complication is even more critical with regard to spine surgery. For example, when a patient cannot be moved suddenly due to an unstable spine, airway management becomes more of a challenge. This needs to be addressed as soon as the patient shows any signs of nausea. Avoiding nausea and vomiting is therefore a matter critical to safety, as prolonged vomiting may cause dehydration and disruption or bleeding of the surgery site.

Researched protocols now rely on grouping patients at risk, based, for example, on previous history, gender, and length of surgical procedure, then matching the group with carefully chosen anesthetic drugs given as part of the anesthetic process. These are given with attention to hydration and oxygenation, and selected antiemetic drugs given intraoperatively. Risk scoring is a relatively new concept [12], thought to be particularly useful.

The most efficient antiemetic drugs in use are the 5-hydroxytryptamine3 inhibitor group, such as granistron and ondansetron, followed by the antihistamines, eg, cyclizine, and dopamine antagonists, such as droperidol and haloperidol. These can be given together to give blanket coverage for high-risk groups. Although it may be impossible to reduce causative factors, with an effective research-based protocol and system in place, risks of nausea, and vomiting are considerably reduced and patient safety and comfort improved.

5   NEUROLOGICAL ASSESSMENT

"The main purposes of the neurological assessment are to detect neurological injury, establish the level of cord compromise, and follow the progression or resolution of the neurological findings" [13].

Performing neurological assessment in immediate postoperative management of all spinal patients is essential as motor function impairment or/and sensory deficit can occur due to nerve damage during surgery. It is important to know the patient's preoperative neurological status, so further impairment or improvement can be detected early.

The actual neurological assessment includes motor function examinations, which aim to test the strength of different muscle groups. Before this assessment can be carried out, the carer must have knowledge of the spine anatomy and the dermatome map (see chapter 1.1 Anatomy of the spine).

The patient will be asked to complete seven physical tasks in which to assess their motor responses, highlighting the levels being tested via the nerve roots.

Physical tasks

- Flex and extend elbows—tests C5 and C7.
- Flex and extend wrists—tests C6.
- Pinch forefinger and thumb—tests C8 and T1.
- Hip adduction or cross the legs—tests L2.
- Flex and extend the knee—tests L3 and L5.
- Flex and extend the ankle—tests L4 and S1.

Muscle power

Muscle power can be graded using a grading scale for muscle strength (**Table 3.7-1**).

Simply asking the patient if they can feel the touch of the examiner's hands performs the sensory observations. Pinprick or catheter tug can be used for the assessment. Sensation should always be assessed against the presence of a nonaffected part of the body, eg, the face of a tetraplegic patient. Any sensory deficits like absent or altered sensation, or the presence of pins and needles, must be reported to the medical staff.

"The level of spinal cord injury is the level at which sensation is altered or absent, or at which weakness or absence of movement is noted. This level may be different from that of the column injury" [14].

Examination of both motor and sensory functions is very important, as the patient may have sensory damage without motor damage and vice versa. Both sides of the midline should be examined individually and compared, because variations can occur.

0	No muscle contractions, complete paralysis.
1	Flicker or trace of contraction.
2	Moves but cannot overcome gravity.
3	Moves against gravity but cannot overcome resistance of examiner's muscles.
4	Moves with some weakness against resistance of examiner's muscles (grade 4 can be described as 4+ if against strong resistance or 4- if against slight resistance).
5	Normal power and strength.

Table 3.7-1

Grading scale for muscle strength.

6   PERIPHERAL DRAINAGE CARE

6.1   RENAL

The surgical patient is at risk of developing acute renal failure. Causes include the following:

- Hypotension—due to the effect of the drugs used during the anesthesia and analgesia, plus blood and fluid loss.
- Hypovolemia—due to blood, fluid and electrolyte loss.
- Sepsis—this causes altered renal hemodialysis in impaired function through immunologic mechanisms.
- General anesthetic—alters renal hemodialysis and can cause hormonal imbalance which leads to disturbed renal autoregulation and compromise of normal renal blood flow [15].

The kidney receives 20–30% of cardiac output. If the patient is hypovolemic or hypertensive, the ability of the kidney to function becomes increasingly impaired. If the renal blood supply remains insufficient, renal hypoxia will occur leading to acute tubular necrosis.

The patient will have their urine measured hourly and is expected to pass 0.5 ml per hour per kg. They should have a mean blood pressure of over 100 mm Hg and an acceptable pulse rate. Cool, pale extremities will also indicate a poor circulating volume. Central venous pressure should also be constantly measured. If there is any suggestion of renal failure, the anesthetist must be informed and the cause of renal insufficiency sought and treated.

6.2   WOUNDS AND WOUND DRAINAGE

Following spine surgery, the patient will have a surgical wound and drain(s) in situ. In recovery, the patient's wound site and drainage bottles must be monitored throughout the duration of their care.

If a rapid saturation of fresh, bright, red blood appears on the wound dressing, there should be no attempt to take it down. Reinforcement with a larger pad and as much pressure as possible may help to prevent a hematoma developing and, more importantly, to prevent contamination of the wound with bacteria. Infection delays wound healing (this topic is addressed in more detail in chapter 3.1 Infection control and preventative precautions in the operating room), and a sudden increase in wound leakage can indicate venous or arterial bleeding. The operating surgeon must be informed allowing a reassessment in case the patient requires reexploration of the wound. The drainage should be recorded on the fluid balance charts and the drains checked frequently to ensure suction is maintained.

6.3   CHEST DRAINS

Anterior thoracic spine surgery patients will have a chest drain in place; this is due to disruption of the pleura. Pleural or thoracic drains remove fluid and air from the pleural space by negative pressure; this aids reexpansion of the lungs.

6.4 WATER SEAL DRAINAGE

The principles of water seal drainage are:

- Underwater seals act as a one-way valve allowing air to be expelled from the pleural space and preventing it from reentering during the next aspiration.
- The system must be kept airtight.
- Collection chambers must be kept below the level of the patient to prevent fluid siphoning back into the patient.
- If possible keep the collection chamber at least 100 cm below the level of the chest, as suction pressures of −80 cm H_2O can occur if breathing becomes obstructed.
- Frothing in the chamber makes measurement of the volume of fluid drained difficult. Reduce frothing by using saline in the bottles instead of sterile water.
- If there is no respiratory swing (oscillation) this indicates the drain tube is obstructed, possibly by blood clots, a twisted tube, the seal no longer being airtight or the lung having been completely reexpanded.
- Clamping a pleural drain in the presence of a continuing air leak invites the formation of a tension pneumothorax.

A stringent delivery of care is required due to the importance of the cavity they are maintaining.

The following aids and observations must be applied:

- Assisting patient into a comfortable position to further encourage free drainage.
- Administering any appropriate analgesia to ensure comfort both at the drain entry point and also on respiration.
- Monitoring and recording all drainage within the water seal system.
- Maintaining fluid in the underwater seal chamber; observe for swinging at all times.

---

7   SKIN AND PRESSURE AREA CARE

This subject is very important throughout all the stages of care for the spinal patient.

The care of skin and pressure points must not be overlooked during the delivery of immediate postoperative care (see also chapter 3.3 Patient positioning for spine surgery).

Postoperatively, the spine surgery patient is at risk of developing pressure sores due to reduced mobility and/or altered sensation. The areas at risk must be checked as soon as possible and regularly thereafter during their stay in recovery. Any areas of concern that have developed during surgery must be communicated to the recovery nurse at handover, to enable continuous monitoring and immediate treatment of any affected sites.

Facial eye edema is commonplace when the patient has been in the prone or knee-chest position on the operating table. The eyes must be observed closely and the patient reassured, as it may be difficult for them to open their eyes fully. The edema is associated with positioning during surgery, and also the excessive amount of IV fluids administered during the procedure.

As soon as consciousness and pain levels allow, the patient may be rolled laterally to check both the wound and pressure areas. Any changes in the skin/wound appearance must be documented for continuity of observation/care on the ward.

Maintaining basic nursing care, especially strict clean and dry bed management, is paramount at all times, as uneven and wet sheets can be the beginning of pressure sores. The correct pressure-relieving mattress must be in situ before the patient is repositioned after surgery.

Pressure points relating to recovery which must be checked are:

- Oxygen masks—ensure they are not too tight over the bridge of the nose (consider nasal prongs).
- Saturation probes—these can easily cause pressure damage on the patient's fingers (rotate regularly).
- Blood pressure cuff—due to high inflation pressures it can cause skin damage, especially in children or the elderly (soft bandage or similar can be applied beneath the cuff).

8   EMOTIONAL AND PSYCHOLOGICAL SUPPORT

When a patient undergoes surgery of any description, psychological and emotional support has an enormous role to play when caring for a patient in recovery [16].

Patients who have had spine surgery often have altered perceptions of body image before the operation due to scoliosis, therefore the nurse needs to be extremely sensitive and reassuring when discussing this issue. Patients often feel very overwhelmed and emotional after a successful surgery has been performed. Patients who are well informed about their spine surgery tend to be less anxious in recovery.

"Another benefit of psychological preparation for back surgery is less pain and less need for postoperative pain medication and also fewer complications to surgery and recovery [17]."

When the spinal patient arrives in recovery they are often still unconscious from the anesthetic. This short phase of recovery allows time for the set up and connection of all the vital and invasive monitoring. Thus, when the patient awakens, the nurse can focus on the emotional and psychological elements of recovery, as well as on demystifying the monitoring equipment, and arterial and central venous pressure lines that are standard practice, as these are frequent sources of anxiety for patients.

Many spinal patients undergoing deformity surgery are under 20 years of age. To reduce anxiety for the patients, parents are encouraged to come into the recovery area. This reassures both the patients and parents that the surgery has gone well. However, this is only allowed when the patients are aware of their

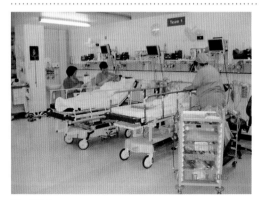

Fig 3.7-1
It is important that patients can develop trust and confidence in the recovery nurse.

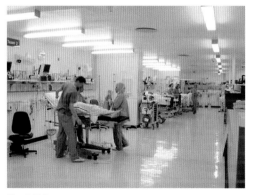

Fig 3.7-2
Immediate postoperative care at the highest possible standard is important.

surroundings and can maintain their own airway, as seeing their child in the immediate postoperative surgery state can be distressing for parents.

Patients need to feel that their circumstances and feelings are appreciated and understood by the recovery nurse without criticism or judgment—if the patients feel that the attention they receive is caring and tailored to meet their individual needs it is more likely that they will develop trust and confidence in the recovery nurse (**Fig 3.7-1**).

Preoperative visiting or assessment clinics are important factors in improving patient outcomes from major surgery. Here, information and reassurance can be given, hopefully addressing some of the anxieties that patients may have about their surgery.

Recovery is the first step to patients achieving a better quality of life following surgery. We as healthcare professionals must do all within our power to ensure the immediate postoperative care is delivered at the highest possible standards (**Fig 3.7-2**).

9   BIBLIOGRAPHY

1. **Hatfield A, Tronson M** (1992) *The Complete Recovery Room Book.* London: Oxford University Press.
2. **Atkinhead A, Smith G** (1996) *Textbook of Anaesthesia.* 3rd ed. London: Churchill Livingstone.
3. **International Association for the Study of Pain** (1992) *Management of Acute Pain: A Practical Guide.* Seattle WA: IASP Press.
4. **Dobson F** (1997) Anatomy and physiology of pain. *J Community Health Nurs (Br);* 2(6):283–291.
5. **Hawthorn J, Redmond K** (1998) *Pain: Causes and Management.* Oxford: Blackwell Sciences.
6. **McCaffery M** (1999) Basic mechanisms underlying the causes and effects of pain. McCaffrey M, Pasero C (eds), *Pain: Clinical Manual.* 2nd ed. CV Mosby.
7. **McIntyre P, Ready L** (2002) Pain Foundation. Week 1. Nursing Times Special Focus. *Nursing Times;* 98(38):41–44.
8. **World Health Organization** (1996) *Cancer Pain Relief.* 2nd ed. Geneva World Health Organization.
9. **Carr CJ, Mann EM** (2000) *Pain: Creative Approach to Effective Management.* London: McMillan.
10. **Nelson TP** (2002) Postoperative nausea and vomiting: understanding the enigma. *J Perianaesth Nurs;* 17(3):178–189.
11. **Brady M, Kinn S, Stuart P** (2004) Preoperative fasting for adults to prevent perioperative complications. *Cochrane Review in the Cochrane Library,* Issue 1, Chichester: John Wiley.
12. **Eberhart LHG, Hogel J, Seeling W, et al** (2000) *Evaluation of Three Risk Scores to Predict Postoperative Nausea and Vomiting.* Oxford: Blackwell Science.
13. **Hirschfeld A** (1990) Emergency room care of patient with spinal cord injury. Alderson JD, Frost EAM (eds), *Spinal Cord Injuries: Anaesthetic and Associated Care.* London: Butterworths. 33–46.
14. **Harrison P** (2000) *Managing spinal Injury: critical care.* Spinal Injuryies'Association.
15. **Montgomery Dassey B, Guzzetta C, Vanderstaay Kenner C** (1992) *Critical Care Nursing.* Philadelphia: Lippincott.
16. **Adams AP** (1994) *Recent Advances in Anaesthesia and Analgesia.* London: Churchill Livingstone.
17. **Deardorff WL, Reeves JL** (1997) *Preparing for Surgery: A Mind-Body Approach to Enhance Healing and Recovery.* Oakland: New Harbinger Publications.

3.8   EMERGING TECHNOLOGIES

1   MINIMALLY INVASIVE SPINE SURGERY

Minimally invasive spine surgery (MISS) has had an unplanned evolution. As other surgical specialties embraced this technology, the scope of MISS, together with its complexity has increased. Smaller incisions give improved patient cosmesis, and visualization is aided, even improved with endoscopic illumination and microscopic magnification. However, it is important to stress that the operation itself remains the same.

The wider use and development of MISS has led to the emergence of a whole array of specially designed instruments, with both hand-held and power-driven derivatives available to be used for smaller incisions, either endoscopically or with microscopic magnification. Video technology and the simple attachment of a camera to the rigid telescope has enabled the entire surgical team to view procedures and pathology on TV. In fact, MISS has changed the operating environment with its complex instrumentation and high-tech equipment. Patient demand has ensured its popularity and it has now become the

method of choice for many surgical procedures. However, it is technically demanding for both the surgeon and operating room personnel (ORP) alike, and there is a definite learning curve required for this type of surgery.

Minimally invasive procedures reduce the incision and in doing so produce minimal soft-tissue and muscle destruction. The importance of this in spine surgery is that the maximal function of the ligaments and soft tissues, which are integral to the normal function of the spine, are retained. In fact, there is no pathophysiological difference between major trauma and a surgical operation [1]. Minimizing the trauma inflicted by the operation lessens the stress response of the body, which is most certainly in the best interests of the patient.

Various surgeons have demonstrated that metabolism, endocrine activity, and immunological responses are significantly lower following minimal access surgery. Small incisions also improve cosmesis, and in time minimal soft-tissue dissection and destruction will reduce operation time and minimize blood loss. Reduction of operative time with minimal soft-tissue destruction in turn improves postoperative pain and recovery, which reduces the length of hospital stay.

The goals of any MISS are identical to those of the open procedure:

- Sufficient decompression of neural structures.
- Stabilization and fusion where appropriate.
- Correction of spinal balance both in the sagittal and coronal planes.
- Correction of deformity.
- Pain relief.

The visualization obtained during endoscopic surgery is particularly advantageous, as it provides a focused illumination, and magnification of the specific surgical field being examined. The use of multiple small portals, particularly with angled lenses, allows a more extensive visualization of the surgical field.

Minimal invasive surgery will continue to grow with improvements in imaging and instrumentation, particularly with the advent of 3-D cameras and virtual reality. This is a progressive technology that has not yet achieved its full potential.

1.1   CLINICAL APPLICATIONS OF MISS

Anterior surgery

This includes laparoscopic assisted surgery, which involves carbon dioxide insufflation transperitoneally, ie, through the peritoneum, or balloon-assisted gasless retroperitoneal dilatation, ie, the peritoneal sac and its contents are moved as a whole out of the way.

Indications for thoracoscopic surgery include:

- Tissue, disc, or bone biopsy.
- Symptomatic thoracic disc herniation (radiculopathy or myelopathy).
- Anterior release and fusion for spinal deformities (rigid scoliosis > 45° on side bend x-rays).
- Rigid kyphosis (> 60° on hyperextension x-rays), anterior release and fusion to prevent crankshaft phenomena in skeletally immature (Risser 0 or 1 maturity, Tanner 0 or 1 sexual status, age < 10 years, open triradiate cartilages).
- Internal costoplasty for rib prominences associated with various types of scoliosis.

Spine surgeries undertaken using such techniques include:

- Lumbar interbody fusion, either minilaparotomy transperitoneal or retroperitoneal approach.
- Transthoracic thoracoscopic surgery (with or without fusion) for disc herniation, tumor or infection.
- Thoracoscopic assisted scoliosis correction.

Posterior surgery

This type of MISS has been practiced for a long time and in general largely involves the use of microscopic magnification or image-guided percutaneous procedures. Indications for microendoscopic discectomy are the same as for conventional microdiscectomy.

Such procedures include:

- conventional microdiscectomy,
- microendoscopic discectomy,
- percutaneous discectomy ,
- laser discectomy,
- intradiscal electrothermal therapy (IDET) practiced percutaneously,
- posterior lumbar fusion with instrumentation,
- posterior lumbar interbody fusion (PLIF),
- transforaminal lumbar interbody fusion (TLIF),
- vertebroplasty/kyphoplasty,
- nerve sheath injection/transforaminal epidurals are other percutaneous procedures, which are dealt with elsewhere.

1.2   DISADVANTAGES OF ALL FORMS OF MISS

For every new surgical technique there are always disadvantages. In the instance of MISS the primary disadvantage is the steep learning curve required to master the techniques. In addition, high-tech equipment is costly and required at the outset so there is a considerable initial cost outlay in terms of both time (training staff in the new techniques) and money.

With thoracoscopic surgery there is an increased:

- dural tear rate,
- potential for spinal cord injury,
- pulmonary complications (hemothorax, pneumothorax, pneumonia),
- intercostal neuralgia (chest wall pain),
- large vessel injury (segmentals, azygous vein, aorta, vena cava),
- poor implant placement.

For scoliosis surgery the disadvantages are:

- suboptimal disc excision,
- pseudarthrosis (nonfusion),
- smaller diameter rods used, possibly leading to implant breakage.

Damage to nerve structures encountered during thoracoscopic surgery include:

- intercostal nerves—during portal insertion or internal costoplasty,
- sympathetic plexus,
- vagus nerve,
- phrenic nerve,
- greater and lesser splanchnic nerves.

Lengthier operative times may be necessary for laparoscopic surgery, especially initially, and a general surgeon may be required to help with the surgical approach. Abdominal distension occurs from carbon dioxide insufflation and there is an increased complication rate involving visceral injury to the:

- stomach,
- small and large bowel,
- kidney, ureter, and bladder.

Vascular injury to the:

- aorta,
- vena cava,
- common iliac artery and vein,
- left iliolumbar vein.

Nerve injury to the:

- nerve root or sympathetic plexus,
- inferior hypogastric plexus injury—retrograde ejaculation in male, vaginal dryness in female.

Mini open laparotomy can be undertaken with the aid of frame-based retraction systems (**Fig 3.8-1a–b**).

The frame provides advantages similar to laparoscopic surgery, but without the necessity of scaling the steep learning curve, and dealing with the inherent challenges involved in using high-tech equipment.

The surgery can be easily performed using a single small incision, leading to overall shorter operative time, comparable complication rates, and rapid patient recovery.

Because of the learning curve for both ORP and surgeons it is important to follow a standard sequential training system. The entire scrub team must attend a course to obtain specific training and certification for the procedure. The team needs to learn pertinent anatomy, indications and inherent complications, and be aware of these during any procedure undertaken.

Appropriate practice on cadavers and animals by both surgeons and ORP will aid the smooth and successful use of high-tech equipment. Visiting an experienced surgeon and team to watch them operate in practice is exceptionally valuable, and so too is performing cases under the supervision of an experienced surgeon.

Patient safety is evidently of primary importance. Following the correct sequence of procedures will help reduce complications during the learning process.

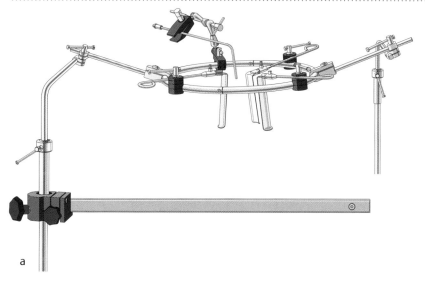

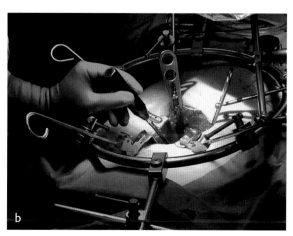

Fig 3.8-1a–b
a Frame-based retraction system.
b Frame in situ.

2   VERTEBROPLASTY AND KYPHOPLASTY

Vertebral body augmentation is a relatively new technique which has made rapid advances over the last 20 years, especially in Europe and the United States. This technique is slowly gaining momentum and acceptance in the UK.

Vertebral augmentation was originally developed to fill voids after tumor resections and as an adjunct to fix screws in deficient bone. Polymethyl methacrylate cement was used and found to be a very stable supportive material following such resections:

- Percutaneous vertebroplasty was first used and developed by Galibert and Deramond et al [2] for the treatment of a painful hemangioma of the second cervical vertebra.
- Percutaneous kyphoplasty was introduced by Reinhardt to circumvent the shortcomings of percutaneous vertebroplasty (PVP) [3, 4].

Since then, the techniques have been developed to treat osteoporotic fractures, spinal metastases, hemangiomas, and osteonecrosis. In particular they are rapidly gaining momentum in the treatment of osteoporotic insufficiency fractures.

PVP is a minimally invasive technique, which involves the injection of bone cement into the vertebral body, under fluoroscopic control, usually via introducers placed through the pedicles (**Fig 3.8-2a–b**).

Kyphoplasty is a similar procedure, however, a balloon is first inflated within the vertebral body, to restore vertebral height and reduce kyphosis, after which cement is placed in the cavity which has been created (**Fig 3.8-3a–d**).

Both techniques have the same objectives:

- relieve pain,
- restore function and mobility,
- strengthen the vertebral body, thereby reducing abnormal movement and potential neural damage.

There is currently no evidence to suggest that kyphoplasty is more clinically efficacious than vertebroplasty.

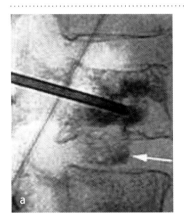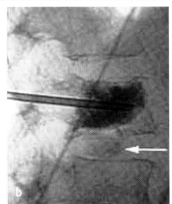

Fig 3.8-2a–b
Lateral x-rays showing a percutaneous vertebroplasty.

Vertebral compression fractures are most commonly due to osteopenia secondary to advancing age. Metastatic disease is a less common but, nevertheless, an important cause of compression fractures and spinal instability. A large population-based study found that vertebral compression fractures were due to osteoporosis in 83%, trauma in 14%, and cancer in 3% of cases [5]. These patients can experience pain, which can be of a varied duration and severity.

The majority of insufficiency fractures are treated:

• conservatively with analgesics,
• by bed rest until the fracture heals,
• by preventative treatment of the osteoporosis and bracing (generally in an extension cast).

Pain usually eases within four weeks to three months using the above approaches. However, a small percentage is left with persistent pain and limited mobility.

Surgical intervention is often difficult in elderly patients with persistent pain and limited function, as the internal fixation systems cannot be adequately anchored and securely fixed in the osteopenic bone. Metastatic disease at multiple levels can also reduce the stability of the construct. This results in high rates of implant failure due to pedicle screw and laminar/pedicle hook pullout. In addition, elderly patients and those with metastatic disease are often not medically fit enough to undergo major surgical procedures. Complication rates are far higher due to their comorbidity and the prolonged operative time required for a secure construct.

Wound healing is reduced in these patients, and bone graft less likely to take. Anterior surgery risks damage to the friable arteriosclerotic vessels, and implant struts such as cages tend to fail as they cut into the soft bone. Hence, augmentation techniques have developed to address these problems.

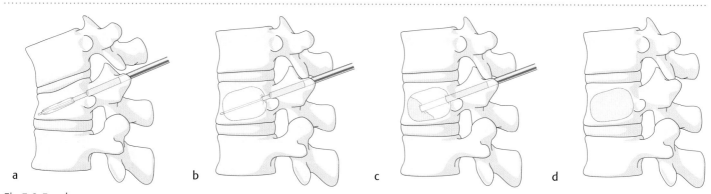

a b c d

Fig 3.8-3a–d
Technique of kyphoplasty.

The results of vertebral augmentation vary depending on the indication, patient selection, operator skills and complication rates. The majority of published results are based on retrospective case series, and there have been very few prospective controlled trials. In general, augmentation for osteoporotic fractures successfully relieves pain in 57–97% and in metastases by 50–91%. Mobility has been shown to improve by 60–100% in patients with osteoporosis.

There have been no published data comparing the cost effectiveness of vertebroplasty or kyphoplasty with conservative management of these patients.

Vertebral augmentation has been shown to increase both the strength and stiffness of the vertebral body and to prevent collapse [6]. The ideal patient with an insufficiency fracture should be neurologically intact with no demonstrable instability and should be referred preferably within four months of injury. Many authors advocate referral only after six to eight weeks of conservative management, as there is often a substantial resolution in pain during this period.

For metastatic disease the pain-relieving effects of radiotherapy can be delayed for up to two weeks, while the effect of bone reconstruction is only partial and can take several weeks.

Vertebral augmentation does not modify the long-term outcome of metastases but it does facilitate more rapid analgesia and early mobility, which is an advantage in these patients. Chiras et al [7] felt that it was helpful in cases of persistent pain following chemotherapy or radiotherapy.

Contraindications to vertebral augmentation are absolute and relative. Absolute contraindications include:

- locally-active infection,
- cardiopulmonary compromise preventing the procedure or fitness for anesthesia,
- coagulopathy,
- neurological signs of cord compression (these may require surgical decompression).

Relative contraindications include:

- lack of definable vertebral collapse,
- collapse < 20%,
- unstable fracture patterns, and those which prevent safe access,
- posterior wall involvement (risks extrusion of cement and canal compromise, but the procedure is still possible if the cement is placed anteriorly under close monitoring),
- epidural extension of metastatic tumor and pedicular involvement,
- pregnancy,
- allergy to cement constituents,
- a small target in inexperienced hands,
- intraoperative difficulty viewing the fracture,
- lack of surgical back-up,
- young age.

2.1 COMPLICATIONS OF VERTEBROPLASTY OR KYPHOPLASTY

Complications occur in 1–5% with osteoporosis, 2.5% in hemangioma and 5–10% in metastases.

The most common complications are:

- cement extravasations resulting in injury to spinal cord,
- nerve root,
- adjacent viscera,
- adjacent level end-plate fractures secondary to stress transfer,
- hemodynamic problems,
- sudden death syndrome from cement polymer reaction,
- fat embolism.

The overall rate of serious complications is very low.

2.2 NICE GUIDANCE

Due to the growing popularity of both vertebroplasty and kyphoplasty the National Institute for Clinical Excellence (NICE) has recently issued guidelines for vertebral augmentation. These are summarized below.

Percutaneous vertebroplasty (September 2003):

- Should be limited to patients with pain refractory to conservative treatment.
- Should be performed only with access to a spine surgery service.
- The performing clinician must have received adequate training to an appropriate level of expertise and, in particular, must follow the manufacturer's advice when mixing the cement to reduce the risk of embolization.
- The main complications, which are uncommon, include damage to neural or other structures due to needle placement or leakage of cement, and infection.
- Pain relief is achieved in 57–97% and a reduction in medications in 50–91%.

Balloon kyphoplasty (November 2003):

- There is insufficient current evidence, and special arrangements for consent, audit, and research must be in place.
- Prior discussion within a multidisciplinary team and with spine surgeons is required.
- Should be limited to patients with pain refractory to conservative treatment.
- The performing clinician must have received adequate training to an appropriate level of expertise and, in particular, must follow the manufacturer's advice when mixing the cement to reduce the risk of embolization.
- The main complications are cement leakage, allergy, nerve or spinal cord damage and infection.

---

3   DISC REPLACEMENT SURGERY

Functionally, the intervertebral disc is responsible for the transmission and reduction of complex spinal compressive, torsional, and bending forces applied during normal physiological loading. Hydrostatic pressure within the nucleus pulposus primarily resists compressive and bending forces, while the annular fibers primarily resist torsion. Approximately 80% of loading occurs anteriorly within disc/end plates and 20% posteriorly within facets and posterior structures.

The close functional relationship that exists between the intervertebral disc and facets is such that facet arthritis rarely occurs without the presence of disc degeneration and that normal disc function appears to be protective of facet function. Disc degeneration occurs when changes within nucleus and annulus occur. Reduction of proteoglycans within the nucleus lowers its ability to bind water and hence withstand compressive loads, resulting in altered disc biomechanics. Reduced collagen, together with alterations to its normal helical structure within the annulus, lowers its ability to withstand torsion. Both of these events result in increased stresses, susceptibility to injury, annular tears, and disc herniation. Pain fibers start to innervate the inner annulus and can cause pain resulting in degenerative disc disease and degenerate disc pain syndrome.

Compression alone does not account entirely for the pain experienced in clinical practice. Pain experienced by patients is complex in its origins. The search in recent years for an understanding of the pathophysiology of sciatica and discogenic low back pain has focused attention on the cellular and molecular activity of the intervertebral disc tissue. It has been shown that degenerate disc tissue from patients with sciatica synthesizes inflammatory cytokines, the quantities increasing with increasing exposure of the nucleus. Disrupted disc tissue has been shown to release inflammatory cytokines such as IL-beta, IL-6, TNF-α (tumor necrosis factor alpha) and other algesic chemicals.

Phases or spectrum of disc degeneration

Phase I: Early degeneration, altered motion segment biomechanics, reduced compressive load bearing capacity. Annular tears may cause pain, disc herniation may cause sciatica.

Phase II: Instability phase, where degeneration progresses, and facet subluxation, increased facet loading, facet arthritis, and segmental instability occur.

Phase III: Hypertrophy of ligaments and osteophyte (bone) formation heralds the body's attempt to stabilize the disc. This can cause spinal stenosis and nerve root entrapment syndrome/sciatica, degenerative spondylolisthesis and scoliosis = lumbar spondylosis

The primary problem with current surgical treatment (discectomy, laminectomy or fusion) is that it does not restore normal spinal function. In fact, it destroys the three joint complexes, and therefore can potentially worsen segmental spinal instability. Further instability can cause increased pain requiring additional procedures, eg, decompression and/or fusion.

With spinal fusion there is a theoretical acceleration of adjacent segment degeneration that can lead to:

- disc degeneration,
- stenosis,
- disc herniation.

These are seen in clinical practice during long-term follow-ups with patients [8].

Combined posterior fusion with pedicle screws is very destructive to posterior soft tissues and musculature. Complications of posterior surgery include:

- nerve root injury,
- dural tears,
- bleeding,
- harvesting bone graft has risks—infection, chronic donor site pain, and fracture.

Goals of disc replacement

The goals of disc replacement surgery are primarily to remove the source of pain, ie, the painful degenerate disc. Once in place the prosthesis will restore segmental disc height, which in turn restores physiological lumbar lordosis and overall sagittal alignment. This maintains and restores normal spinal segmental motion and therefore protects adjacent segment degeneration. With the restoration of disc height the facet joints are off loaded and facet arthritis prevented. Disc replacement may also indirectly decompress the neural foraminae.

Patient selection

Patient selection criteria are strict. Firstly, the patient must present with back pain secondary to one or two level degenerative disc disease, which has failed six months of the usual conservative modalities.

The MRI must show early disc degeneration (less than 50% collapse) with or without positive discogram. If a discogram is not undertaken then the presence of high-intensity zone and/or end plate inflammatory changes are highly suggestive of discogenic pain. It is usual for the patient to receive discography as confirmation of their pain source in their preoperative workup [9].

Examination must reveal normal neurological status. There must be no evidence of advanced facet arthritis on MRI (CT scan optional).

There are relative contraindications, which are previous discectomy or laminectomy (facets preserved), and spinal stenosis.

Absolute contraindications include:

- spinal deformity,
- gross spinal stenosis,
- infection,
- metabolic bone disease, eg, osteoporosis or osteomalacia,
- fractures,
- absent posterior elements, eg, spondylolysis or spondylolisthesis,
- previous facetectomies,
- congenital bony anomalies and poor psychological profile with abnormal pain diagrams.

3.1   TYPES OF DISC REPLACEMENT SURGERY

There are two basic types of disc replacement currently available:

- nucleus replacement (**Fig 3.8-4**),
- total disc replacement surgery or arthroplasty (**Fig 3.8-5**).

The arthroplasty is comprised of two cobalt-chromium alloy metal end plates with an ultra high molecular weight polyethylene core or liner. Primary stability is achieved by anchoring the metal end plates to the vertebral end plates by means of teeth or metal keel. Secondary stability occurs when bony ingrowth occurs into the titanium plasmapore-coated end plates.

Ideal design of disc arthroplasty

Ideally the components are manufactured with biocompatible materials, which have superior endurance, ie, excellent metal and polyethylene wear characteristics, since most patients are young. The prosthesis must maintain and restore normal spinal segmental motion:

- flexion and extension,
- lateral bending and rotation,
- restore segmental disc height,
- lordosis and global saggital profile.

There are two types of prosthesis; constrained and semi constrained. The prosthesis is constrained in an attempt to avoid instability and dislocation, particularly of the polyethylene insert. The degree of constraint remains controversial. The metal end plates must have optimal immediate and long-term bony fixation.

Early results of current prospective studies show significant reduction in immediate postoperative pain and recovery but no difference in clinical outcome compared to AP spinal fusion.

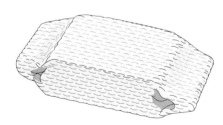

Fig 3.8-4
A nucleus replacement.

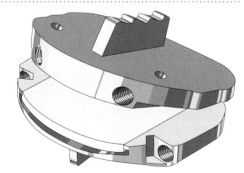

Fig 3.8-5
A disc replacement.

Surgery for disc arthroplasty

Preoperative planning is of prime importance when choosing correctly sized components. This may include optional preoperative spiral CT scan of spine. MRI or CT angiography is useful to look at large vessel bifurcation and hence to plan the operative approach. Dual energy x-ray absorptiometry is required if there is concern about osteoporosis. There should be a backup team with a vascular or general surgeon available, with a laparotomy tray ready in case of open conversion because of the risk of vascular injury. A nasogastric tube to empty the stomach and an urinary catheter to empty the bladder away from the surgical field is required to aid the surgical approach.

The technique involves:

- An anterior approach, which can either be retroperitoneal, or transperitoneal (indicated in those with previous laparotomy).
- Image intensification is needed throughout the procedure for location and exact placement of the prosthesis in both the AP and lateral planes.
- Precise positioning of prosthesis in both frontal and sagittal planes under fluoroscopic guidance is of paramount importance.

Once the disc space is exposed, complete removal of the nucleus with a complete posterolateral release is needed. This may require removal of posterior annulus and osteophytes for optimal annular balancing/tensioning. The cartilaginous end plate is removed.

3.2   COMPLICATIONS

The complications for disc arthroplasty are the same as for anterior spinal fusion:

- abdominal wall hernias,
- vascular injuries,
- visceral injury,
- nerve injury—nerve root or sympathetic plexus,
- inferior hypogastric plexus injury—retrograde ejaculation in males, vaginal dryness in females,
- dural tears,
- bleeding—epidural plexus.

Complications specific to the prosthesis are:

- migration,
- dislocation or subsidence of prosthesis,
- malpositioning of prosthesis in the long term may cause asymmetric facet loading leading to facet arthritis and facet joint pain.

Factors leading to failure

Patients should be screened to exclude any factors which could lead to failure. Patients with advanced facet arthritis, for example, will fail due to their secondary facetal pain; patients with osteoporosis may fail as the prosthesis has an increased risk of subsiding. Inadequate disc clearance will result in poor positioning of the prosthesis. If sufficient clearance and releases are not undertaken advanced disc degeneration or collapse will lead to malpositioning of the prosthesis and early failure.

Controversies

It has been argued that the increased risks of anterior surgery may not be justified in view of equivocal results with posterior fusion. Poor results occur if facet degeneration is present. There are only relative short- to medium-term results on clinical outcome, and the long-term effects of polyethylene wear and metal debris on adjacent spinal nerve roots are not yet known.

4   DYNAMIC STABILIZATION SYSTEMS FOR THE SPINE

Intervertebral disc degeneration is a contributing factor to low back pain and may be partially ascribed to abnormal loading patterns on the disc. The usual approach to tackling discogenic back pain is to excise the fragment of herniated disc where compression is a problem or to restrict the motion of the spine at the degenerative or painful level. Today this usually involves fusion, with or without rigid spinal instrumentation.

Discectomy removes the neural compression causing the pain but increases mobility and decreases the rigidity of the motion segment. Discectomy only treats the consequences of discal degeneration. Fusion on the other hand, while it provides pain relief, restricts mobility and significantly alters the loading environment of the disc in question as well as the adjacent disc away from the ideal physiological state. Fusion is also a therapeutic dead end. You cannot mobilize a motion segment, ie, reverse a fusion once one has been undertaken.

Flexible fixation devices were therefore designed (**Fig 3.8-6**) to treat the cause of discal degeneration, ie, instability, and to provide spinal stabilization while allowing a physiologically advantageous load through the disc. Dynamic stabilization has emerged once more as a treatment for discogenic low back pain. The goal of this type of system is to treat discogenic pain while preserving mobility and restoring stability. It also keeps options open for further treatment as these systems can later be converted to fusions. Aims of dynamic stabilization systems:

- to provide pain relief,
- to preserve the mobility of the segment instrumented,
- to maintain the physiological loading status of adjacent segments as much as possible.

How do these dynamic systems work?

Dynamic systems are said to preserve the disc when the patient's normal stabilization systems, ie, muscles, ligaments, and the disc itself, have failed. It has been claimed that these systems not only buy added time for the degenerate level, but also contribute to disc cell healing. Dynamic implant cadaver mechanical studies show that with these systems in situ both rigidity and stability are increased. The stiffness of the segment is seen to increase, whilst segment displacement decreases. There is a transfer of the load towards the posterior arch, which reduces intradiscal stress. Hence, the disc of the instrumented level supports no more load than the intact disc. This encourages healing in the problematic segment, and, advantageously, adjacent segments are less likely to have problems as the behavior of these levels is not altered.

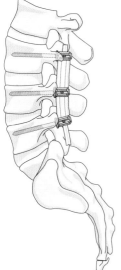

Fig 3.8-6
A dynamic stabilization system.

5 BIBLIOGRAPHY

1. **Troidl H** (1990) The general surgeon and the trauma surgeon- binding the wounds. *Theor Surg;* 5:64–74.

2. **Galibert P, Deramond H, Rosat P, et al** (1987) [Preliminary note on the treatment of vertebral angioma by percutaneous acrylic vertebroplasty.] *Neurochirurgie;* 233:166–8.

3. **Coumans JV, Reinhardt MK, Lieberman IH** (2003) Kyphoplasty for vertebral compression fractures: 1-year clinical outcomes from a prospective study. *J Neurosurg;* 99:44–50.

4. **Lieberman IH, Dudeney S, Reinhardt MK, et al** (2001) Initial outcome and efficacy of "kyphoplasty" in the treatment of painful osteoporotic vertebral compression fractures. *Spine;* 26(14):1631–1638.

5. **Cooper C, Atkinson EJ, O'Fallon WM, et al** (1992) Incidence of clinically diagnosed vertebral fractures: a population-based study in Rochester, Minnesota, 1985–1989. *J Bone Minor Res;* 7:221–227.

6. **Grados F, Depriester C, Cayrolle G, et al** (2000) Long-term observations of vertebral osteoporotic fractures treated by percutaneous vertebroplasty. *Rheumatology;* 39:1410–1414.

7. **Chiras J, Depriester C, Weill A, et al** (1997) [Percutaneous vertebral surgery. Technique and indications.] *J Neuroradiol;* 24(1):45–59.

8. **Kumar MN, Jacquot F, Hall H** (2001) Long-term follow-up of functional outcomes and radiographic changes at adjacent levels following lumbar spine fusion for degenerative disc disease. *Eur Spine J;* 10(4):309–313.

9. **Bertagnoli R, Kumar S** (2002) Indications for full prosthetic disc arthroplasty: a correlation of clinical outcome against a variety of indications. *Eur Spine J;* 11:S131–136.

GLOSSARY

GLOSSARY OF SPINAL TERMS

Achondroplasia   A common form of congenital dwarfism.

Active mobility   A range of motion patients can perform under their own power.

Adolescent scoliosis   A spinal curve that presents after puberty, but before maturity.

Adult scoliosis   A spinal curve that presents after skeletal maturity.

Angiography   An opaque liquid, injected to highlight blood vessels when x-rayed.

ALIF   Anterior lumbar interbody fusion; the surgical procedure wherein the disc is surgically replaced with cages or allograft.

Allograft   A tissue or organ transplanted from a donor. Within spinal surgery it is usually freeze-dried bone from a cadaver or freshly frozen donated femoral heads.

Ankylosing spondylitis   Rheumatoid arthritis of the spine. Also known as "Bamboo Spine", due to the bamboo shoot-like appearance seen on an x-ray.

Ankylosis   A joint that no longer moves or has little or no motion.

Annular bulge   An early stage of disc degeneration.

Annular tear   A tear in the outer tough ring of the disc.

Anulus fibrosus   A ring of fibrocartilage surrounding the intervertebral disc.

Anomaly   A malformation usually caused by a congenital or hereditary defect.

Anterior body   Solid anterior section.

Anterior discectomy and fusion   Surgical removal of the disc, which is then replaced with an allograft or autograft and implants may or may not be applied.

Anterior disc herniation   Protrusion of the nucleus pulposus.

Anterior longitudinal ligament   Attached to the base of the occipital down to the sacrum.

AP   An x-ray view where the beam passes from the anterior to the posterior.

Apex   The most extreme point.

Apical vertebrae   The vertebra with the greatest distance from the midline.

Aplasia   The congenital absence of a structure.

Aponeurosis   A flat sheet of connective tissue which joins muscle to bone or bone to other tissue.

Arachnoid   Membrane of the spinal cord.

Arthrodesis   Surgical immobilization of a joint (fusion).

Arthropathy   Disease of the joint.

Articular   Of or pertaining to a joint.

Articular process   Two processes on each side of the vertebra that articulates with adjoining vertebra.

Articulate   To join by means of a joint.

Aseptic   No bacterial contamination.

Asymptomatic   No symptoms.

Atrophy   The wasting of muscle tissue.

Autograft   A tissue or organ transplanted within the same body. Within spinal surgery it is usually iliac crest bone, or rib.

Avascular   Inadequate blood supply.

Bending x-rays   X-rays of the extension and flexion of the spine, routinely taken before surgical correction of deformities

Bifid   Split in two.

Bifurcation   A site at which any given structure divides in two.

Bilateral facet dislocation   A cervical injury with extensive ligamentous destruction.

Block vertebrae   Congenital fusion of two adjacent vertebrae with no motion.

Bone graft   The use of bone in spinal fusions.

Bone spur   An overgrowth of bone following injury.

Brachial plexus   A network of nerves in the lower cervical and upper thoracic spine.

Brooks fusion   A C1–C2 posterior fusion, with iliac crest bone secured with wires.

Burst fracture   A comminuted vertebral body fracture with bone fragments in the canal, where both the superior and inferior end plates are usually fractured.

Canal stenosis   Narrowing of the spinal canal.

Cancellous bone   Inner structure of bone make-up.

Capsule   A fibrous and ligamentous tissue that encases a joint.

C-arm   A portable image intensifier.

Caudal epidural   An epidural injection through the sacral hiatus.

Cauda equina   The roots of the upper sacral nerves and at the termination of the spinal cord, usually at L1 vertebrae in the form of a bundle of filaments within the spinal canal, resembling a horse's tail.

Cauda equina syndrome   Pressure on the nerves in the lumbar region causing nerve root irritation. Can lead to loss of bowel and bladder control.

Caudal or caudad   Distally or downward towards the feet.

Cephalad or cranial   Superior or upwards towards the head.

Cerebral palsy   Birth injury/defect affecting the control of the motor system.

Cerebrospinal fluid   Fluid in which the brain and spinal cord reside, circulating in the arachnoid space.

Cervical collar   A cervical protector which wraps around the neck and is available as a soft or hard product.

Cervical rib   An extra rib found in the cervical spine.

Chance fracture   An unstable fracture which involves a horizontal disruption which travels through the vertebral body, the spinous process and the neural arch.

Clivus   Skull base bone.

Cloward procedure   A surgical technique for anterior cervical discectomy and fusion.

Cobb angle   A method used to measure the degree of scoliosis on an AP x-ray.

Coccygectomy   Surgical removal of the coccyx.

Comminuted   More than two fragments.

Compression fracture   The collapse of the vertebral body.

Concave   Rounded, depressed surface.

Congenital scoliosis   A structural deformity caused by an irregular or distorted vertebra.

Convex   Rounded, elevated surface.

Congenital   Existing at or dating from birth.

Conus medullaris   Where the cord tapers at the L1 segment.

Corpectomy   Excision of vertebral body.

Cortical bone   The dense outer surface of bone makeup.

Costal cartilage   The cartilage that connects the rib to the sternum anteriorly.

Costotransversectomy   Surgical procedure used to excise laterally a herniated thoracic disc.

CSF   Cerebrospinal fluid.

CT   Computed tomography.

Debridement   Surgical removal of dead or damaged tissue from a wound.

Decompression   Surgical procedure to relieve pressure on the spinal cord and nerves.

Decubitus   A horizontal patient position.

Degenerative disc disease   Deterioration of the chemical and physical makeup of the disc space.

Degenerative scoliosis   A lateral curvature of the spine caused by advanced degenerative disc disease. This causes the destruction of the articular facets and deformity within the vertebral body.

Dens   Part of C2. Can be known as the odontoid peg.

Dermatome   The distribution of the sensory nerves near the skin responsible for pain, tingling, and other sensations.

Discectomy   Surgical procedure to remove the intervertebral disc.

Disc herniation   When the nucleus of the disc ruptures.

Discitis   Inflammation of the disc.

Discogram   A local procedure conducted under imaging to show the structure within the disc.

Discopathogenic   Abnormal function of the disc.

Disc space   Area between two vertebrae.

Distal   Furthest from the point of reference.

Distraction   Parting of the joint surfaces by traction.

Double curve   The development of two major curves, equal in size in scoliosis, usually found in patients with neuromuscular diseases.

Dura   The outer covering of the spinal cord.

Dural tear   CSF escaping from the dural sack. This can occur during surgery.

Durotomy   An opening in the dura.

Dysraphism   A failure of the posterior elements to fuse around the spinal cord, eg, spina bifida.

Eggshell procedure   A surgical fracture of a vertebra so it can be collapsed and removed.

Elephant man's disease   A hereditary disorder that affects the nerves. 50% of the time this disease is related to scoliosis.

End plate   A layer of cartilage at both ends of the vertebral body approximately 1 mm in depth.

Epidural abscess   Infection localized in the epidural space.

Epidural injection   A steroid injection into the epidural space, usually in the lumbar spine for pain relief.

Epidural vein   A large valve-less vein, part of the internal vertebral venous plexus which drain the spinal cord, CSF, and spinal canal.

Erector spinae muscles   A group of muscles found in the lumbar spine.

Facet   A flat anatomical surface.

Facet block   A steroid injection into the facet joints, usually in the lumbar spine for pain relief.

Facet dislocation   A cervical spine injury, may be either unilateral or bilateral.

Facetectomy   Surgical removal of all or a part of a facet joint.

Facet hypertrophy   Enlargement of the facet joint due to degeneration.

Facet Joint   A synovial joint found at the posterior of each vertebra.

Facet rhizolysis   A local procedure to destroy the nerves to the facets, to treat lumbar pain.

Fascia   A fibrous structure separating one body compartment from another.

Foramen   A small opening or hole.

Foramen magnum   The opening in the base of the skull through which the spinal cord passes.

Foraminotomy   Removal of overlying bone to enlarge the foramen.

FRA   Femoral ring allograft.

Friedreich's ataxia   An inherited degenerative disease associated with the nervous system.

Fusion   Surgical immobilization of a joint.

Gallie fusion   A surgical technique for posterior fusion using wires on C1 and C2.

Gardner-Wells tongs   A device in which to apply skeletal traction to the cervical spine.

Halo   A device used to immobilize the cervical spine.

Hangman's fracture   A fracture in the lateral masses of C2.

Harlow wood bone biopsy trephine   Biopsy needle used to obtain small cores of bone.

Hemisacralization   Congenital fusion of L5 to the sacrum, but only on one side.

Hemivertebra   An incomplete development on one side of a vertebra.

Herniated disc   A defect in the annulus allowing leakage of the nucleus pulposus, commonly known as a "slipped disc".'

HNP   Herniated nucleus pulposus. Another term for a "slipped disc".

Hyperkyphosis   A curve that presents more posterior than a normal kyphosis.

Idiopathic   A disease or condition with an unknown cause.

Idiopathic adolescent scoliosis   The most common form of scoliosis. Presents as a lateral curve with malformed vertebral bodies.

Iliac apophysis   The end plate which runs along the wing of the ilium. Used to estimate skeletal growth remaining for scoliosis.

Iliac crest   The superior point of the ilium, commonly used to harvest material for autografts.

Ilium   The superior and the principal of three bones of the lateral half of the pelvis.

Impingement   A compression of two structures, entrapping the organ or tissue it houses.

Infantile scoliosis   A lateral curve that develops before the age of three years.

Inferior   An anatomical region, below the area being discussed.

Inion   Bony prominence at the back of the skull.

In situ   Accepted or original position.

Interbody fusion   A surgical procedure replacing the disc space with autograft or allograft.

Intercostal   The space between each rib.

Interspinous ligament   The ligamentous attachment that connects adjoining spinous processes.

Intervertebral   Area between two neighbouring vertebrae.

Intraspinal   To be found within the spinal canal.

Ipsilateral   Meaning the same side.

Jamshedi needle   A small core needle used for tissue biopsies.

Jefferson fracture   A cervical fracture of C1. It usually presents as a four-part fracture resulting from a direct blow to the head.

Juvenile scoliosis   A deformity which occurs between the ages of 3 and 10 years.

Kyphosis   A natural curve of the thoracic spine.

Lamina   A broad shield of cortical bone forming part of the neural arch.

Laminectomy   A surgical procedure for removing the lamina.

Laminotomy   A surgical removal of part of the lamina.

Lateral mass   A section of the cervical spine to which the vertebral artery travels.

Ligament   Tissue which connects two articular surfaces.

Ligamentum flavum   A ligament found in the posterior surface of the spinal canal, from the axis to the sacrum.

Lordosis   A natural curve of the cervical and lumbar spine

Lysis   A slip forward of the vertebrae.

Magerl screw fixation   A surgical procedure for a posterior lumbar fusion.

Major curve   The largest of a two-curve scoliosis.

Marfan syndrome   A connective tissue disease.

Mastiod tip   Bony prominence behind the ears.

Medulla oblongata   Brain stem.

Meninges   The three membranes covering the spinal cord.

Meningitis   Inflammation of the meninges.

Meningocele   A imperfection in the neural arch of the vertebral body.

Microdiscectomy   A small incision surgical procedure with little tissue disturbance for a HNP.

Moe technique   A posterior surgical fusion of the facet joints.

Morphology   The science of the structure and form of organisms.

Motion segment   Two adjacent vertebrae that move against each other.

MRI   Magnetic resonance imaging. An imaging procedure detailing both soft tissue and bone anatomy.

Myelogram   A contrast injection into the subarachnoid space in the lumbar spine.

Myelopathy   Disorder and pathological changes in the spinal cord.

Myeloradiculitis   Myelopathy plus inflammation of the nerve roots.

Neoplasm   A cancerous growth.

Nerve root   A collection of fibers that exit the spinal cord at every level.

Nerve root canal   The opening where the nerve root exits the spinal canal.

Nerve root decompression   A surgical procedure to release pressure from a nerve root.

Nucleus pulposus   The gel-like substance found in the vertebral disc.

Nerve root tethering   When a nerve root is stretched over a stationary object.

Neuroblastoma   Malignant growth.

Neurogenic claudication   A clinical symptom associated with lumbar central canal stenosis.

Neurologically intact   No disruption of the spinal cord.

Oblique   A radiographic image used regularly to find the "Scottie dog sign".

Occipital   The back of the skull.

Odontoid fracture   A fracture of C2.

ORIF   Open reduction and internal fixation.

Ossification   A process of forming bone.

Osteoblast   A bone-forming cell.

Osteoblastoma   A benign tumor of the spine, usually found in the posterior elements.

Osteoclast   A bone cell.

Osteophyte   A bone overgrowth found around a joint area and post-injury site.

Osteoporosis   A mechanical failure due to a decrease in the bone density.

Osteotomy   A surgical procedure for cutting bone.

Paget disease   A metabolic disease of bone which affects the spine.

Paraplegia   Paralysis of the lower half of the body which involves both legs.

Pars   A point of reference between the superior and inferior facet joints.

Pathological fracture   Collapse of the vertebral body due to osteolytic destruction and neoplasm.

Peanut   A small solid swab used for tissue dissection in surgery.

Pedicle   The mass of bone for screw fixation when using implants.

Percutaneous   A surgical procedure performed through the skin without tissue destruction caused by surgical incisions.

Periosteum   The membrane covering the bone

Pia mater   A vascular membrane of tissue around the spinal cord.

PLIF   A surgical procedure for a posterior lumbar interbody fusion.

Poliomyelitis   An acute virus affecting the anterior horn cells of the spinal cord.

Posterior longitudinal ligament   Attached to the posterior base of the occipital down to the coccyx.

Proximal   The closest point of reference.

Pseudarthrosis   A failure to obtain a solid fusion postoperatively.

Quadriplegia   Paralysis of both the arms and the legs.

Radicular   Originating from the nerve root.

Radiculalgia   Pain associated with the nerve roots.

Radiculopathy   Pathological condition associated with the nerve roots.

Ramus   Branches of nerves.

Retts Syndrome   A genetic disorder mainly affecting girls which causes mental retardation.

Retroperitoneal   Area behind the posterior layer of the peritoneum.

Rib hump   The ribs are enhanced due to the vertebral rotation on the convexity of a spinal curve.

Risser sign   A method to measure skeletal maturity.

Sacroiliac arthrodesis   A surgical procedure to fuse the S1 joint.

Sacroiliac joint   The area where the sacrum and the iliac bones form a joint.

Sacrum   The tail end of the spinal column.

Sagittal curve   One of three curves present in the normal adult spine.

Sagittal plane   A division of the body into right and left parts.

SCAAPF   Simultaneously combined anterior and posterior fusions.

Scheuermann disease   A deformity of the spine which presents from the age of 10–13 years as inflammation of the bone and cartilage.

Sciatica   Pressure on the nerves in the spinal canal or pelvis.

Scoliosis   A deformity of the spine which affects both the rotation and curve asymmetry. Can present from infancy to adulthood, and is the commonest form of spinal deformity.

Scottie dog sign   In an oblique x-ray of the lumbar spine the posterior elements take on the form of a Scottish terrier.

Sepsis   The presence of infection.

SMK   A radio frequency probe.

Soft-tissue injury   A traumatic injury to the muscles, tendons and ligaments.

Solid fusion   When the surgical fusion procedures have been successful and a bone mass has formed, showing no movement between the vertebra bodies.

SPECT scan   Single photon emission computed tomography scan.

Spina bifida   A congenital defect of the lumbosacral region.

Spinal canal   The bone space that protects the spinal cord.

Spinal cord   The longitudinal cord of nervous tissue that extends along the spine.

Spinal shock   A short-term paralysis due to suppressed reflex activity, which follows spinal cord trauma.

Spondylitis   Inflammation of the vertebrae.

Spondylolisthesis   A forward displacement of a vertebra overshadowing its distal partner, usually in the lumbar spine.

Spondylosis   A degenerative disease caused by the process of aging.

Stenosis   A narrowing of the central canal.

Subdural space   The space below the dura.

Subluxation   A partial dislocation.

Subperiosteal dissection   Removal of tissue from bone.

Supraspinous ligament   Found at each end of the spinous processes from C7 down to the sacrum.

Superspinous ligament   A ligament which is attached to the spinous processes.

Sympathetic chain   Nervous chain running along either side of the spinal cord.

Teardrop fracture   A fracture of the cervical spine.

Thecal   The dura covering the cauda equina.

Thoracolumbar junction   The area of the spine from T12–L1.

Tomography   An x-ray technique to examine thin sections of bony structures.

Translaminar fixation   A surgical procedure to form a fusion with facet screw fixation.

Vertebra   One of twenty four bones which make up the spine.

Vertebral artery   A posterior artery in the neck supplying blood to the spinal cord.

Vertebrectomy   Removal of vertebral body   anterior.

Wake-up test   Slight reduction of the anesthetic agents, allowing the patient to wake up enough to respond the commands.

Wedge fracture   A compression fracture affecting the vertebra due to the collapse of the anterior wall.

Whiplash injury   A sprain or strain of the cervical spine muscles and ligaments due to a hyperflexion injury.